I0109792

A LAND
NOT
FORGOTTEN

A LAND
NOT FORGOTTEN

Indigenous Food Security & Land-Based
Practices in Northern Ontario

EDITED BY MICHAEL A. ROBIDOUX
AND COURTNEY W. MASON

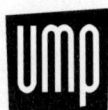

UMP

UNIVERSITY OF MANITOBA PRESS

© The Authors 2017

25   24   23   22   21   3   4   5   6   7

All rights reserved. No part of this publication may be reproduced
or transmitted in any form or by any means, or stored in a database
and retrieval system in Canada, without the prior written permission
of the publisher, or, in the case of photocopying or any other
reprographic copying, a licence from Access Copyright,
www.accesscopyright.ca, 1-800-893-5777.

University of Manitoba Press
Winnipeg, Manitoba, Canada
Treaty 1 Territory
uofmpress.ca

Cataloguing data available from Library and Archives Canada
ISBN 978-0-88755-757-6 (PAPER)
ISBN 978-0-88755-517-6 (PDF)
ISBN 978-0-88755-515-2 (EPUB)

Cover and interior design by Jess Koroscil
Cover image: Simeon Cutfeet, an Oji-Cree community member who lives
in Wapekeka, northwestern Ontario. Photograph by Courtney W. Mason.

Printed in Canada

This book has been published with the help of a grant from the
Federation for the Humanities and Social Sciences, through the Awards
to Scholarly Publications Program, using funds provided by the
Social Sciences and Humanities Research Council of Canada.

The University of Manitoba Press acknowledges the financial support for
its publication program provided by the Government of Canada through
the Canada Book Fund, the Canada Council for the Arts, the Manitoba
Department of Sport, Culture, and Heritage, the Manitoba Arts Council,
and the Manitoba Book Publishing Tax Credit.

Funded by the Government of Canada   Canadä

CONTENTS

ACKNOWLEDGEMENTS

This collection would not have been possible without the strong partnerships that were formed over the many years of working with First Nations communities and organizations in Northwestern Ontario. These partnerships were originally fostered with the assistance of Margaret Kenequanash, the executive director of the Shibogama Tribal Council, to whom we are extremely grateful. We are deeply indebted to the leadership at the Nishnawbe Aski Nation (NAN) who originally partnered with the Indigenous Health Research Group (IHRG) in 2006, and have continued to support our work ever since. In particular, we would like to thank Wendy Trylinski at NAN for her continued involvement in IHRG research activities and for facilitating relationships with NAN communities.

There are so many people to thank at the community level, starting with the chiefs and band councils from the Kasabonika Lake First Nation, Wapekeka First Nation, and Wawakapewin First Nation. In each of the communities there are hunters, food preparers, and food champions who were instrumental in all aspects of our community involvement. This not only meant working with researchers to achieve project goals, but taking us into their homes, sharing food, sharing knowledge, sharing culture, sharing time, taking care of our students, and generally providing life-changing experiences for all of us. We are forever grateful to Clara Winnepetonga, Derek Winnepetonga, Chris Anderson, Jonas Beardy, Laura Semple, Irene Semple, Keith Mason, Leon Beardy, Cathy Pemmican, Simon Frogg, Arlene Jung, Archie Meekis, Rhoda Meekis, and Leighton Anderson.

We would also like to thank the many research coordinators and research assistants, whose work was critical throughout the various stages of research for this project and in the manuscript preparation. Thank you to Shinjini Pilon and Corliss Bean for their patience and perseverance in managing IHRG research activities and all of the partnerships that came along with the research. Thanks to our wonderful students who lived and worked in communities throughout the project, Michelle Kehoe, Melanie St-Jean, Meagan Ann Gordan, Rebecca Brodmann, Desirée Streit,

Cindy Gaudet, Michael Padraig Leibovitch Randazzo, and Erin O'Reilly. We would also like to thank Caroline Anna Head for her assistance formatting the manuscript.

We are grateful to the editorial staff at the University of Manitoba Press, who have been extremely patient with us as we put this book together. In particular, we would like to thank Glenn Bergen, who first approached us about this book project; Jill McConkey, who was great throughout the whole process; and Barbara Romanik for her diligent and thoughtful editing. We, along with Simon Frogg's family, are indebted to Glenn and Jill for arranging for a preliminary version of the book to be sent to Simon just days before his passing. It meant so much to Simon to see his words in print. Thank you.

As always, we need to acknowledge our families for their ongoing support. Sharon, Sarah, and Hannah, thanks for looking out for one another while Michael was away. Courtney wishes to thank Josephine, his parents, and his family for the many ways that they support his work.

This book was made possible by a financial contribution from the Social Sciences and Humanities Research Council of Canada and Health Canada, through the Canadian Partnership Against Cancer.

Prologue

CONVERSATIONS WITH WAWAKAPEWIN ELDER SIMON FROGG

Over the last decade, through our community-based research, we have had the great honour of working closely with Oji-Cree Elder Simon Frogg. Our relationship with Simon has significantly informed our understandings of the connections between food, the well-being of people, and the environment. In sharing with us his experiences and traditional teachings, Simon has helped us to see the connections between our work and Indigenous ways of knowing. In Oji-Cree culture, there is virtually a story for every type of food. These stories, often told with a humorous tone, contain directions for respectful interactions with other living beings as well as cautionary warnings for breaching our responsibilities to one another. At Simon's request we share with you the story of Wesakechak and the Geese.

Simon Frogg: You ask me where we need to start this book project? Well, when we started to work with the University of Ottawa, I said if we're going to be talking about food and how it's supposed to help the well-being of our people, I have to know where this is based—if there is any connection to our way of understanding. That's what I'm interested in and how we arrived at that connection. What I have come to realize is that the perspective of our people, or what we believe, can be found in the teachings that have been handed down, primarily through what are fostered in the legends. For me that's always a good starting point. For instance, when I have to deal with some type of process or program or whatever, the first thing I do is try to figure out where it exists in our teachings, in the legends. That is the first thing I try to do. I try to find if there is some type of original direction relating to whatever I'm doing. It starts with the historical aspects of traditional foods and how they are gathered. We have a long history shaping how we understand these things, which have been made known to us through the legends and stories associated with them. So my suggestion is that we include portions of those in the book, stories that tell this history, the knowledge of our traditions, and our teachings around wild foods. The securing, preparing, and storing of wild food—there are characters in the legends that give us knowledge and teachings that go far back in time. It's not something we just pulled out of a hat. It's something that our people understood through teaching stories and legends, which have been handed down to us. There's so many of them. There's virtually a story for every food source. Of course there is a component of humour, but they are made up of different characters, characters from a divine period when there were only animals. Do you remember the Wesakechak story? That's also a prophecy, do you remember?

Wesakechak and the Geese

Wesakechak is a humorous character. He's also scary in a lot of ways. The story begins with Wesakechak having killed some geese. So he roasted them in the sand. But he had the feet sticking up from the sand so he would know where they are. Then he built a fire over that. But then he got sleepy, so he asked his rear end to watch out for him while he slept so that no one would steal his geese. But then some people showed up so his rear end woke him up the first time and told him that there were some people in the bushes. He looked around and he couldn't see anyone. He got angry at his rear end saying there was no one there and to not wake him up if there's no one there. This happened a second time. And he got angrier still when he didn't see anybody and scolded his rear end again. And then it happened a third time, but his rear end didn't wake him up. So those people came out and pulled his geese out of the sand . . .

stuck the feet back in and took off with the geese. The whole
thing about this is the humour associated with him having
the conversation with his rear end and him getting angry.
Because when he finds his geese stolen, he is angry again
at his rear end and says "Why didn't you wake me?" And
his rear end responded, "Well I did, but you got angry at
me." But this only made Wesakechak even more angry. So
he rubbed his rear end on the coals of the fire. This caused
scabs to start forming from the burns on his rear end and
then he wiped those scabs on the rocks . . . they fell off
and they remain on the rocks. And that's when he said the
prophecy: "In the future, when there is no food, our people
will be able to eat this." The scabs are the lichen that is on the
rocks, which was important for people's survival.

The reason why this story is told, aside from the fact that it's funny, is
that it speaks of a prophecy about a time when food will be scarce. People
in the past, they knew how to survive and knew what to look for and what
to use. This is what this story is about, but it is also interwoven with other
longer stories. It prophesizes that in the future there will be no food, so our
people will need to take what is left on the rocks in order to survive. Those
"scabs" from Wesakechak's ass contained all the vitamins and minerals.
When we were young, old people collected the lichen from the rocks, and
they crushed it. Then they mixed it into the food that they were preparing—
especially into stews. So that's an actual process that people [went through]
when I was child; I was actually shown this. Even though I didn't understand what prophecies were, at some point in time I was told the legend and
that is how I connected those ideas. But this isn't really done anymore in
terms of transferring knowledge. But I guess I'm doing it now, I'm relaying
it in a professional way—I guess I am doing that [laughs].

Wesakechak is an important character for a lot of reasons. As a universal character he shapes the holders of the story, shapes who they are as
a people. He's the foolish one, the foolish character. And the predominant
aspect of the foolish character is that it is humorous, meaning that we can't
take ourselves seriously all the time. We have to utilize the fun part, the

humorous part, of who we are and what we do. So that's one aspect of it. Now the other aspect of Wesakechak is that he is involved in shaping, in laying out what will happen in the future. Part of this process involves the land itself as the people who share these stories have the actual representations, geographical representations, in their territory that make up the legends.

An example of that is way up north, up in Fort Severn. The earth cracked. So what Wesakechak did, he stepped over it—he was a giant—he stepped over the crack. And his first step was into Big Trout Lake. There's an island there. And the island is called Wesakechak's Stepping Stone. So there's a round rock on that island. But inside that rock is sort of a cave, and that's referred to as Wesakechak's Stepping Stone. His next step was into Big Beaver House. And why is it called Big Beaver House? There's a shape there, a hill that looks like a beaver house. And in Wunnumin there is the beaver dam, you know, where the water backs up. That is because Wesakechak killed a beaver, one of the giant beavers. He continued upstream and there's a place where he ate the beaver and there's a big pot there in the middle of the rapids. So that's how those types of stories are geographically influenced. They are actual representations of the legend and the geography itself. That's the other aspect of them. That's why I say Wesakechak stories are interwoven into other stories or other parts of the legend as is the character himself. They teach us what our people need to do and the prophecies are interwoven into all the stories. So if you're talking about food, you may wish to consider it, you know about starvation and the Windigo stories—they are primarily metaphors for starvation. They serve different purposes. But one of the things that people don't really understand is that they are teaching too. People often overlook the fact that they are teaching, teaching about what not to do—you never go into a state of starvation. That's why they are told this way.

One of the interesting aspects about learning from the legends, especially the Windigo legends, is to try and make an analogy to understand the meanings, like the metaphor of starvation. I like to compare them to how pilots are trained. They are trained to get out of spiral dives, out of spins. To get out of the spin you need to perform three actions almost simultaneously. Now you do this at 5,000 feet above ground when you're being trained. So basically when a plane is in a spin, or a dive, it's not flying anymore, it stops flying. You as a pilot need to make it fly again by the three actions. But the thing is, the reason why the pilots are taught this in training is, so they never get themselves into this spiral state. So similarly with the Windigo legends, they are told so that people never get into that state of starvation. The stories are told over and over again, for the same reason the pilot learns to get out of a spin, so that the people know what to do to avoid a bad state.

Everything is interrelated . . . in terms of how people exist, and how the earth is related with each other through relationships to the land. And likewise how people have always looked after themselves. It's a holistic way of looking at everything . . . it starts from the phases of the earth, and then likewise the phases of life. An example of this is how the earth has been created after the great flood. There were certain animals that were involved in getting a piece of earth and the earth was developed from that. That's a story that our people were aware of, the value of planning. You had to be able to plan. That's what those teachings in the legends, that's what they teach, that's what they tell—what the animals did, what they were involved in. So we take the humans then. They took the lessons from those [animals], and they started inhabiting the world that they saw because you have to understand that there were different levels of existence. First you have [the period] when only the animals were around. They were involved in setting the behaviour, or things that needed to be done on an ongoing basis. And different animals, according to their capabilities, did such and such. And when the humans came, they took those teachings, they used them, and they moved forward with that. And that's how those teachings have been used all this time. And we're trying to [use them still]. There are so many things now out there, with technology . . . even people from Ontario going to Mars, and stuff like that [laughs]. But our knowledge and our teachings still hold—what we were told, what we tell in those stories, and the systems associated with them. Like, the beliefs systems still tell us who we are. In other words, we have something that we believe in. It's just as valid as a Christian set of beliefs, at least equal to, or we can use both at the same time. And it shouldn't make any difference. The only way it will make a difference is if someone gets hardheaded and says that's impossible, you cannot do that. That's based on your belief in a certain way.

You ask the question of what have we lost in having been misled? To me, that is referring to what was removed, or maybe not intentionally, but it amounts to the same thing. That is what was destroyed, that way of doing things. In a different order, in a different way of introducing things. And that has taken a long time for people to realize that all has not worked properly. European ways of life haven't worked well enough, so now we have to take back what we had and start building on what had worked for us in the past. And one of the ways to do this is to begin to try and integrate everything into what we're doing. I think it's important that we teach our people who we are, and the ways that our people survived and lived in the past, our parents and grandparents and so forth. And by learning, our people, they will know who they are and what their history is—what our people were capable of doing. And it is really important for them to know this so they can teach their children the same way. It helps with building identity—knowing who they are—and to instill into them that it is very important to keep this knowledge alive. That's how we view it. We are of the land. The thing, though, is we haven't been informed of how and why that is.

Today, there are so many people my age who don't teach their children and use our language. Children start by learning English as opposed to their own language. It is very important to teach children their own language, not just English. It took several years, several decades, observing this to learn about the impact the loss of language was having on our culture, and that we needed to take steps to try and reverse this impact. By doing cultural activities and having children involved in them—in their language—is one way to help preserve the language. If the language is maintained, then other things will be easier to maintain. I'm not saying that people have to converse only in their own language because we are in a culture that uses English as a medium of speaking but it's extremely important that children, especially ours, speak their own language and know English as well. And it's easy. It's just maintaining that history, and especially integrating the history of the area and of the land along with the history that is being taught in the schools today because our history is like a history outside history. . . . Schools don't really teach the real history of who we were and how we were integral to what happened to this land and to the processes that we were involved with, like contact with the missionaries, the traders, and with the government. It is so important that the proper history of our people can be brought forward along with everything else kids need to learn in school.

You know our prophecies told us that this all was going to happen. That these different people would show up, which is exactly what happened. That had been prophesized. The other thing is that we already had a world view. We already had an understanding of how we were supposed to relate to everything—with every other being, or everything that we're a part of as a people. So we already had a certain order. We understood how we would honour agreements amongst ourselves. In other words, we had agreements, we had arrangements, we had treaties you could say. So we understood those already. And so for us, for our people, that's what they thought they were doing when they entered treaties with Europeans. They agreed on something. They agreed on the meaning of what they believed, what is referred to as the spirit and intent is what they believed. . . . Obviously they wouldn't presume to understand what was written on the treaty, because they couldn't read English to start off with. But they understood the nature of making arrangements and the honour associated with it—in other words the spirit and intent. That's the difference from what I understand happened during the treaty-making process. Essentially it was a different way of thinking about what a treaty meant. The governments of the day, especially during the Victorian era—the Victorian way of thinking was totally different from how our people understood life. And that was brought into the treaty-making process, the Victorian perception of things. That's how it was manipulated, the way the treaty was negotiated, not between the governing parties and the Aboriginal people, but between the provincial and federal governments. They negotiated the treaties between themselves first. And once their treaties were made, the commissioners said they couldn't change the terms of the treaty; they just had to get the people to sign it, to agree to it. In doing so, the white man, the government, changed our relationships with each other and with the land.

As a result of these treaty relations, Aboriginal peoples have been taken advantage of and have not been given what the government promised them. This led to us losing our way of life and our land. What we are doing now is trying to put in place a process to reclaim our culture and our spirituality. The Elders have a lot of information and experience that need to be passed on to people. We're limited by the time we set aside to do these things. The Elders are growing old and they must pass on the knowledge they have. We're talking about this now, about the land, the community, the principles, and the directions. I will tell you what my personal vision is as an Elder in the community. The first thing I want to do is to ensure that spirituality is a key element in our lives. Our people have accepted Christianity from way back. Our forefathers decided that it was the best way for us, but the thing is—our people have been here for thousands of years before Europeans were. Our people believed in the creator and in god and they lived according to what they understood about that. Then with contact, a new religion, Christianity, was brought to them and they accepted it because they believed it was true and it was good. So that's what happened; we are Christian people now. My parents brought me up as a Christian. Their wish was to make sure that we would keep and maintain Christianity and that's what we had to do and we'll maintain that.

However, because of all my experiences and the education I've received, the research I've done and everything else, I know the process and the manner in which this transition occurred was all wrong. I know that the spirituality in our lives today is not correct because some of the teachings about our culture are not correct. My vision is to make sure that all the ceremonies and everything that our people used to do is reintroduced for the future generations of our people. You know like drumming and smoking a pipe. . . . I believe that if this is done properly, we will end up with better Christian people in the future. That is what I believe. Right now, part of our culture and our history has made people reluctant to bring this out . . . so people are not proud of who they are or how they were. For me, that's one of the key aspects in terms of what I want to do. The very important thing about all of this is that we cannot abandon our cultural life, especially our life related to our land and its resources. We have to preserve the spiritual aspect of all of that. If we don't have a spiritual base, in terms of what we believe in, we will not be able to do this. We need to rely on this completely.

COURTNEY W. MASON AND MICHAEL A. ROBIDOUX

Introduction

FOOD SECURITY IN RURAL INDIGENOUS COMMUNITIES

Canadians often learn about food insecurity and related health consequences through international news. Media reports fill television screens
with stories from around the globe of food shortages caused by drought,
flooding, or climate change (Wiebe and Wipf 2011). In Canada, many of
us first learn about food shortages by participating in local food drives and
food banks (Power 2011). These discussions in the news and in everyday
life tend to focus on the economic hardship of *some* families in mostly urban locations, rather than what is problematic with our food policies. Few
explanations are provided as to which communities are disproportionately
affected and why such inequalities exist in our food systems.

Despite national coverage of the pressing issues in Indigenous communities, most urban Canadians rarely consider food insecurity and how
it impacts the health of many people across the country. In particular, why
rural Indigenous communities are vulnerable is not clearly understood by
the general Canadian public. Due to the privileged position of individuals and the general wealth of our nation, few think about where their food
comes from and in what conditions it was produced or processed. This is
related to the massive rural depopulation that occurred in Canada, primarily after the Second World War (McKay 1994). In 1950, almost 40 percent
of Canadians were still classified as living in rural areas. By the turn of the
twenty-first century, only 20 percent of the nation's citizens remained rural

(Statistics Canada 2010). This drastic shift, in where Canadians lived and worked, facilitated an increasing distance, both figuratively and geographically, between urban Canadian consumers and the rural regions where much of their food was grown. This distance has ensured that there is a lack of knowledge about the conditions under which our food is produced and the links between food and health. However, there is a growing interest in these issues even though our food systems are more complex and troubling than most Canadians recognize. Local food movements, farmers' markets, and growing awareness of organic production symbolize the changes that are afoot, but these movements remain mostly the concern of an educated upper middle class, rather than a mass movement that extends across the Canadian public (Hansen 2011).

To increase food security and improve health indicators for all Canadians, a re-evaluation of our food systems, in ways that account for policy, trade, as well as cultural and environmental factors, is necessary.[1] Although this is a daunting task that requires critical perspectives on governmental and industrial power relations at federal and international levels, efforts are being made in localized contexts. Despite the barriers, local food sovereignty movements, especially those that connect to and benefit from broader alliances, are making fundamental differences in the lives of many people across the country and the world.[2] Rethinking our food systems not only decreases reliance on foods from great distances, but also expands our knowledge about, and control of, food sources and networks (Wiebe and Wipf 2011). Public engagement, resistance to current options, and generating alternatives are all factors in changing food systems. These issues are being addressed within broader national organizations such as Food Secure Canada, Nutrition North Canada, the People's Food Policy Project, and others. As a consequence, there is a great deal of optimism about the possible alternatives arising in communities across the country. Localized movements that seek to generate some of their own solutions to food insecurity, increase food sovereignty, and address related health issues are complementing broader national developments.

Although the focus of this book is on Canada, and in particular on Indigenous communities of Northern Ontario (see Figure 0.1), the food and health issues examined will resonate with rural peoples across the country and Indigenous communities around the world that have encountered, or are currently managing, similar challenges. As this book will demonstrate, Indigenous communities have a significant role to play in transforming food systems in Canada and around the world.[3] This is in part because Indigenous communities have an extended history of survival on the land, which included developed food systems and networks. Throughout Canada, Indigenous groups engaged in diverse land-based practices that made use of local or regional ecosystems, fluctuating climates, and varying access to resources, including seasonal patterns of mammal and fish migrations. As Secwepemc scholar Dawn Morrison notes: "For thousands of years, Indigenous peoples have developed a wide range of traditional harvesting strategies and practices, including, hunting, fishing, gathering, and cultivating a vast number of plants and animals in the fields, forests, and waterways" (2011, 97).[4] The development of unique sets of knowledges about diverse ecosystems is the result of millennia of Indigenous experiences engaging in these practices. These land-based practices also included agricultural production in many communities.

Originally these practices and the related knowledges were coveted by early European explores and settlers in North America. They relied upon the generosity of Indigenous peoples and the wealth of their knowledge to understand regional ecosystems in order to survive in harsh environments. However, as this book will show, Indigenous food systems were systematically eroded. This began with the formation of British and French colonial governments and later continued under the Canadian nation state. The change occurred through shifting policy, new economies, and the degradation of Indigenous cultures as well as ways of knowing (Snow 2005). Since colonization, Indigenous peoples have witnessed an erosion of the health and integrity of Indigenous cultures, ecosystems, and social structures that are essential to maintaining their lands and food systems (Alfred 2009). As the following chapters will reveal, environmental degradation, neo-liberal approaches to trade, loss of access to traditional lands, the collapse of tribal political structures, and socio-economic marginalization have all greatly impacted the ability of Indigenous communities to respond to their needs for healthy and culturally relevant Indigenous food and food systems (Morrison 2011).

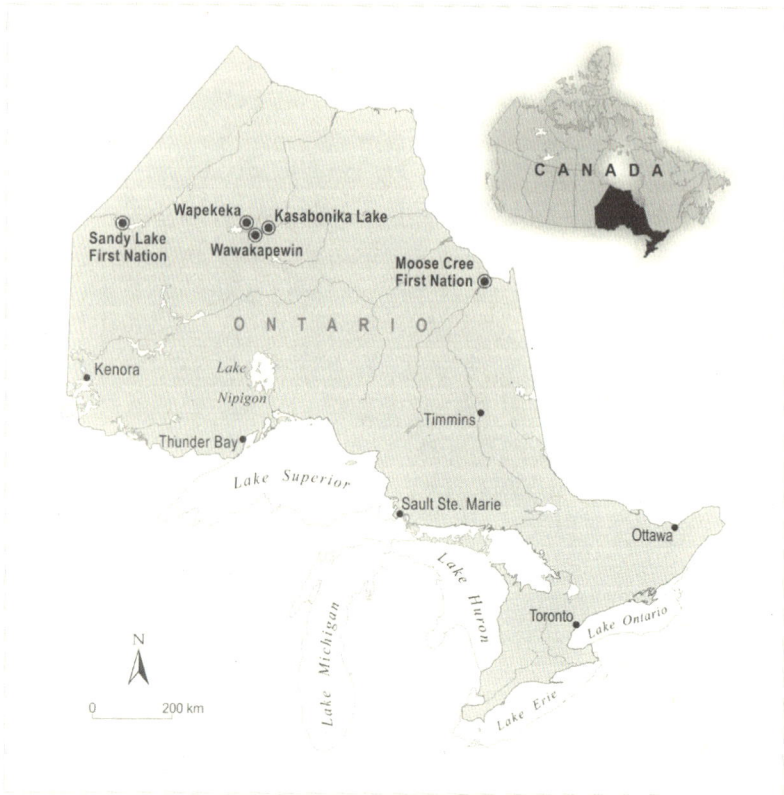

Figure 0.1. Ontario community map. This map identifies the names and locations of the five northern First Nations communities that are profiled in this book. Design by Weldon Hiebert; based on map by Sarah Simpkin, University of Ottawa GSG Centre.

In addition to the historical consequences of colonialism, the barriers that rural Indigenous communities face, to improve access to healthy food, also involve contemporary governmental policy decisions. The failures of governments at all levels to recognize the challenges Indigenous communities encounter and to form policy to address these issues are a major problem. For example, in 2014 a United Nations (UN) envoy, led by Special Rapporteur on the Rights of Indigenous Peoples James Anaya, reported on the situation of Indigenous peoples in Canada noting significant disparities between non-Indigenous and Indigenous peoples in virtually every socio-economic category and health indicator. In a damning statement, Anaya

(2014, 6) writes: "It is difficult to reconcile Canada's well-developed legal framework and general prosperity with the human rights problems faced by Indigenous peoples in Canada, which have reached crisis proportions in many respects." Two years earlier a UN envoy, led by Special Rapporteur on the Right to Food Olivier De Schutter (2012), specifically identified that Indigenous peoples in Canada were three times more food insecure than non-Indigenous Canadians. The UN report was dismissed by the federal government with former Health Minister Leona Aglukkaq saying that De Schutter was an "'ill-informed' and 'patronizing' academic who is 'studying us from afar'" (CTV News 2012). These are only two examples of the federal government's systematic denial of the glaring inequalities that exist within the nation state.

These reports confirm what Indigenous communities and organizations have been claiming for decades. Researchers have also documented the challenges Indigenous peoples face, in particular around food access and the subsequent health problems related to insufficient and low-quality food sources. Indigenous peoples are experiencing an alarmingly high prevalence of obesity (Popkin, Lu, and Zhai 2002) and suffer from a much higher burden of chronic disease than non-Indigenous peoples in Canada (Young et al. 2000; Dyck et al. 2010; Green et al. 2003). The federal government representatives might have scoffed at the UN reports, but they *were* well aware of the gross inequities and the seriousness of the challenges being managed by Indigenous communities. The solutions to redress these issues are not easily conceived nor implemented. While the previous Conservative federal government, and specifically former prime minister Stephen Harper, was more hostile to consider new relationships and less willing to take any meaningful action on these pressing issues, it was simply on a long list of federal governments that have failed to respond to the growing food access and health problems in many Indigenous communities. There is certainly some cautious optimism about the current Liberal federal government, including the new prime minister Justin Trudeau, who appears to have a more nuanced understanding of the problematic relationship between levels of government and Indigenous peoples; however, social, education, and health issues persist and it will be very difficult to address them in the short term. What is notable in this context is that at the community level, land-based practices and Indigenous food systems are currently at the centre of these discussions.

Academics have arguably fared no better than politicians on this front. Despite millions of dollars of research funding allocated to reduce and prevent chronic disease in Canadian Indigenous communities, levels of chronic disease, in particular type 2 diabetes and cardiovascular disease, are increasing (Haman et al. 2010; Young et al. 2000). While it is necessary to recognize that these issues are present and are posing serious health problems for Indigenous communities throughout Canada, more importantly there is a need to provide practical solutions. This book offers potential ways to effectively respond to the complexities of Indigenous health and food systems through a community-derived and -driven approach. This process emphasizes the fundamental relationships between people and the land—what has been lost, and ultimately what is being, or needs to be, restored.

In 2006, the Indigenous Health Research Group (IHRG) was formed at the University of Ottawa. The group comprises multidisciplinary academics from diverse fields such as nutrition sciences, physiology, education, ethnology, toxicology, geography, history, and health sciences. The multidisciplinary approach enables IHRG researchers to appreciate the complexity of Indigenous health issues, which are historically informed, culturally diverse, and impact the physiological health of people in myriad ways. The IHRG utilizes methods that are informed by anthropological traditions and a broad array of clinical and fundamental sciences. Researchers live in particular communities in their attempts to comprehend complex issues such as dietary disease from cultural and biomedical perspectives. This approach enables researchers to understand that dietary disease is not merely a matter of diet, but also a matter of the many factors contributing to food access and food intake of people in their unique cultural, socio-economic, and environmental conditions. Having said this, for researchers working within the field of Indigenous health, it was not immediately apparent how to enact a community-based approach, nor was the approach easily implemented once we fully understood it. Despite a high level of engagement in the theoretical and methodological debates around community-based research, our group has undergone a long learning process to fully appreciate what is truly involved in community-directed action research and the commitment required to live up to the expectations and obligations of this type of work.

Part of this learning curve was to understand how to attain the necessary funding to carry out our research into Indigenous health and food security in Canada. To access funding, researchers need to design projects with questions or objectives that are novel enough to receive positive attention from peer reviewers and that will lead to innovative contributions or publications in their field. Researchers also respond to calls for proposals advertising funding in targeted areas; for example, obesity prevention research. Consequently, research is largely directed by where funding dollars are allocated and what the scholarly community deems valuable. Far too often, these decisions do not actually consider community needs or issues. Since the formation of our group, we have been highly successful in securing significant funding envelopes (with Health Canada's National First Nations Environmental Contaminants Program, Social Sciences and Humanities Research Council of Canada, Canadian Institutes of Health Research, and the International Development Research Centre) and in producing publications in leading journals. While this success has led to our own academic advancement, facilitated the training of students at multiple levels, and fostered strong relationships with community partners, it has rarely translated into sustained changes at the community level.

Despite these shortcomings, the research that was conducted over this period, to address the targeted health and food security challenges, was instrumental in a number of ways. First, it was critical to developing formalized partnerships with Indigenous communities and organizations. Through extensive fieldwork in Indigenous communities, our team was able to build rapport and trust with community leaders and members, gain knowledge of local cultural practices, and deepen our perspectives to appreciate the health challenges many communities face. This was all fundamental to understand how local cultures and environments inform food systems that impact community health. Second, these funding programs allowed us to assemble the right multidisciplinary team capable of drawing from diverse expertise. This was essential to comprehending the food and health concerns of many community members and in documenting eating patterns (Robidoux et al. 2012), levels of chronic disease (Imbeault et al.

2011), and the impacts that environmental contaminants have on local diets (Seabert et al. 2014). Lastly, and perhaps most significantly, these funding opportunities and related research elucidated our limitations as researchers to actually effect change, at least in the manner we initially conducted our projects. We had always characterized our research as community-based because we were working directly with Indigenous peoples in their communities to address observed health issues from their perspectives—in this case, the growing prevalence of chronic disease as well as food insecurity. But it was not until a funding opportunity was presented to us through the Canadian Partnership Against Cancer (CPAC) that we began to more fully appreciate what community research is and how moving beyond research could begin to achieve the results communities envisioned when they first began to work with us.

The CPAC funding was developed through an innovative program called Coalitions Linking Science and Action for Prevention (CLASP). This program was specifically designed to take chronic disease prevention efforts beyond the realm of research and isolated projects, and to bring researchers, policy makers, practitioners, and community members together across multiple jurisdictions. The funding was meant to enable policy makers and practitioners to put research evidence to use in their own domains. For academics, at least in our case, it was an opportunity to see how research could be put into action and to work with communities to develop what they believed were the best practices to address their community's needs. For example, it was apparent from the research we conducted with Indigenous communities in Northern Ontario that people did not have regular access to nutritious foods and that alternative solutions to the high-priced store foods needed to be developed. It was also clear that harvesting land-based foods was difficult, in part, because of the expenses associated with it and gaps in cultural knowledge. We identified through these experiences of working with Indigenous communities essentially what they already knew—that the lack of proper nutrition was having deleterious effects on their health, and that establishing ways to improve their daily dietary intake was necessary to address these health concerns.

Research funding is not typically provided to support communities in forming strategies and programs that respond to the challenges they have identified and that research has corroborated. CPAC's innovative funding model offered the opportunity to put in place targeted evidence-based strategies to respond to chronic disease prevention needs. It enabled our group to work with Indigenous partners to develop the land-based programs they believed would best suit their needs. This collaborative model has since been the driving force of our research group and the basis for fostering our relationships with diverse Indigenous community partners, in multiple provinces and territories throughout the country. This new approach is also what has prompted this book, which has been a work in progress over the past five years. It is a direct result of the multi-sectoral and multi-jurisdictional programs we have formed during the process with Indigenous communities, governmental partners, and policy makers.

This collection emphasizes that there is an incredible amount of cultural diversity in Indigenous communities in Canada, but there are also shared world views, values, and beliefs that underlie their relationships to their territories and the food systems that sustain them. Improving Indigenous health, food security, and sovereignty means reinforcing practices that build resiliency in ecosystems and communities. As the contributors to this book contend, this includes facilitating productive collaborations and establishing networks of Indigenous communities and allies to work together in promotion and protection of Indigenous food systems. Such collaborations will influence diverse groups and bring recognition to the complexity of colonial histories and the destructive impacts on communities. As the following chapters will show, it is our view that acknowledging these histories is a key aspect contributing to change in communities as well as at broader governmental and policy levels.

Overview

This book is divided into five distinct chapters and a conclusion. Each chapter examines certain aspects of Indigenous food security and particular community health issues in the context of Northwestern Ontario. The region, which is north of Lake Superior, is made up of approximately forty First Nations communities, most of which are fly-in, meaning they have no permanent road access. The Ojibwa, Oji-Cree, and Cree populations live in reserves, permanent settlements defined by the Indian Act and "negotiated" under Treaty 9. The expansive region is part of the boreal forest, and is filled with lakes and rivers, which remain critical for transportation and access to the rich wildlife that makes up a considerable part of local diets. The communities, which range in population from forty to just under 2,000, are quite isolated, geographically, politically, and culturally. Situated just south of the 60° latitude, the region is described as subarctic and oddly falls outside of much of national arctic discourse and programming. For example, the Northern Contaminants Program, a program designed to monitor environmental contaminants in local food sources, only focuses on regions north of 60°.[5] The rural communities in this region also face tremendous health concerns, in part due to their isolation and the limited health care services available to them. The Nishnawbe Aski Nation (the territorial political organization that represents Treaty 9 communities) and the Sioux Lookout First Nations Health Authority declared a "public health state of emergency" in 2016 (Gignac 2016). The region has been largely neglected and lacking in public services. As a consequence, communities are experiencing high rates of chronic diseases, suicide, unemployment, and a host of other health as well as socio-economic indicators that are amongst the highest in the country. Despite this, Indigenous communities in this region remain intimately tied to their culture, to their language, and to the land. The land binds people together and remains critical to their survival, in particular as it relates to food security. It is in this sense that the land is *not forgotten,* as it is the cornerstone of Indigenous food systems and Indigenous identities. It is in this spirit that we have assembled this book. Our main objective is to provide a more complete picture of the complexity of health issues Indigenous communities are encountering in this region and how land-based cultural practices are being used as avenues to wellness. Importantly, there is a focus on the response to these challenges at grassroots levels. This includes the partnerships Indigenous people are establishing to enact the changes they want to see in their own communities.

In Chapter 1, Joseph LeBlanc and Kristin Burnett analyze the current issues of food insecurity in Indigenous communities in Northern Ontario by acknowledging the significant historical disruptions to Indigenous food systems. The authors have engaged in community-based action research in multiple Indigenous communities in Northern Ontario over the last decade. In the chapter, they contend that the many efforts to alleviate food insecurity in Indigenous communities have been largely unsuccessful due to an ignorance of the colonial conditions that have extraordinarily altered regionalized food networks. LeBlanc and Burnett not only define how the terms of food security and sovereignty are engaged with in this book, they also explain why rural Indigenous communities continue to especially suffer from the cumulative impacts of deliberate disruptions to their food and political sovereignty. Pointing to both the vulnerability and resiliency of remote Indigenous communities, this chapter outlines some of the difficult decisions Indigenous communities face regarding access to healthy food and local food procurement programs.

In Chapter 2, Francois Haman, Bénédicte Fontaine-Bisson, Shinjini Pilon, Benoît Lamarche, and Michael Robidoux examine some of the issues around the high levels of chronic disease, specifically obesity and obesity-related disease, in Indigenous communities of Northern Ontario. These co-authors profile how the profound and rapid dietary and lifestyle transformations in the region have contributed to the alarming rise in obesity and obesity-related diseases, in particular type 2 diabetes mellitus. Genetics alone cannot explain such a high prevalence of obesity and type 2 diabetes in some Indigenous communities. Clearly, the tremendous challenges they face in relation to food access are major contributors to the high prevalence of chronic diseases. This chapter first problematizes the idea of Indigenous peoples' genetic predispositions to chronic diseases and then presents the current research on the important role played by certain foods in promoting or preventing these diseases. Finally, the authors touch on the complexities of sustaining traditional or healthy food habits in isolated Indigenous communities in Northern Ontario.

The focus in Chapter 3 switches to the communities themselves and to the types of on-the-ground activities taking place to address the transitions communities have endured and the consequential health implications of these transitions. Michael Robidoux describes the IHRG's community-based interdisciplinary approaches, projects, and the group's relations with Indigenous communities in Northwestern Ontario. He asserts that IHRG's community-based research highlights the many health disparities Indigenous people in this region encounter and the multiple factors contributing to these disparities. Robidoux discusses the significant historical impacts that colonial relations and policies have had on Indigenous peoples, in particular on local food systems and the uptake of chronic disease. Utilizing an economic lens, he stresses how increasingly difficult it is for communities to gain access to land-based foods. Derived from the insights acquired by collaboratively working with Indigenous partners in co-designed, land-based programming initiatives, Robidoux draws attention to the considerable successes of numerous projects, but also emphasizes the need to develop and integrate wider food strategies and related programs that address broader food security and health issues.

In Chapter 4, Desirée Streit and Courtney Mason centre on the challenges rural Indigenous communities face in establishing land-based educational curriculum. The authors review the colonial influences that disrupted learning processes in Indigenous communities across the country by providing a brief history of the infamous residential school system. The focus is not only on how schools impacted education and health in Indigenous communities, but also on the ways in which individuals and communities responded to these changes. Following the historical context, the chapter stresses the ways in which some Indigenous communities are reclaiming control of their education systems through land-based curriculum development. Streit and Mason draw from their experiences participating in local food harvesting gatherings in Wawakapewin, a remote Oji-Cree community in Northwestern Ontario. The barriers to and opportunities in designing and implementing Indigenous land-based learning programs are discussed and a curriculum model is provided to demonstrate how community needs can be met while also satisfying provincial curriculum standards.

Chapter 5 builds on the discussion of how and why communities are re-establishing land-based programs for their youth. Cindy Gaudet provides an interesting case study of Moose Factory, an isolated Cree community in Northern Ontario. Relying on interviews with community members and her involvement in developing contemporary land-based programs, she reveals some of the factors that motivate community champions to reconnect youth to the land. By emphasizing the dual purpose of the programs, to transmit cultural knowledge of the land and to promote local food procurement, this chapter provides insight into how the relationships between human, plant, animal, and spirit life are reflected in traditional knowledge and practices. Importantly, the chapter emphasizes the critical role of women, including their leadership and practical skill sets, in the development of land-based programs.

In the conclusion, Mason and Robidoux draw attention to some of the more innovative steps that Indigenous communities are taking, throughout Canada. A few have addressed issues of food security by investing in programs that also improve general health and support cultural continuities. The authors also point to some of the productive collaborations that have developed between Indigenous communities and non-Indigenous organizations. Mason and Robidoux's objective is to demonstrate how communities are responding to local issues and the ways in which they are successfully finding partners to support community-driven initiatives. While the authors identify the barriers Indigenous people continue to face, they also centre on the possibilities that do exist and on what needs to be undertaken in the immediate future to achieve the aspects of food security and sovereignty that critically impact education, health, and broader sustainability issues at the community level.

Notes

1. We borrow from the World Health Organization's definition of food security for a general understanding of the concept. Food security exists when all people at all times have access to sufficient, safe, nutritious food to maintain a healthy and active life. This includes both physical and economic access to food that meets people's dietary needs as well as their food preferences (World Health Organization 2015). A detailed discussion of how we engage this concept throughout the book is explained in Chapter 1.

2. La Via Campesina's definition of food sovereignty, which was coined in 1996, is commonly used. "Food sovereignty is the right of peoples to healthy and culturally appropriate food produced through sustainable methods and their right to define their own food and agriculture systems. It develops a model of small-scale sustainable production benefiting communities and their environment. It puts the aspirations, needs and livelihoods of those who produce, distribute, and consume food at the heart of food systems and policies rather than the demands of markets and corporations. Food sovereignty now appears as one of the most powerful responses to the current food, poverty, and climate

crises" (La Via Campesina 2015). How the concept of food sovereignty relates to Indigenous food sovereignty in rural Canada will be discussed in Chapter 1.

3. Currently in Canada, "Indigenous" has been established as one of the most useful terms for referring collectively to First Nations, Métis, and Inuit peoples. For this reason, throughout the book we have chosen the term when describing general Canadian contexts. However, it is critical to invoke an Indigenous nation's own self-appellation whenever possible and we do this throughout, for example by referring to Oji-Cree peoples. Attention to such terminological specificity prevents a homogenization of distinct cultures and recognizes the heterogeneity and diversity of Indigenous languages and cultural groups (Mason 2014).

4. Indigenous food can be defined as food that has been harvested, prepared, preserved, shared, or traded within the boundaries of respected cultural territories based on values of interdependency, respect, reciprocity, and responsibility (Morrison 2008).

5. Health Canada eventually created a smaller program called the Northern First Nations Environmental Contaminants Program to fund contaminant research south of 60°.

References

Alfred, Taiaiake. 2009. "Colonialism and State Dependency." *Journal of Aboriginal Health* 5 (2): 42–60.

Anaya, James. 2014. *Report of the Special Rapporteur on the Rights of Indigenous Peoples, A/HRC/27/52.* August 11. New York: United Nations General Assembly, Human Rights Council.

CTV News. 2012. "Feds Dismiss UN Envoy's Findings on Hunger, Poor diet." 16 May. http://www.ctvnews.ca/feds-dismiss-un-envoy-s-findings-on-hunger-poor-diets-1.824015.

De Schutter, Olivier. 2012. "Achieving the Right to Food: From Global Governance to National Implementation." In *The Mandate of the Special Rapporteur on the Right to Food.* 17 October. United Nations: Special Procedures of the Human Rights Council. http://www.fao.org/fileadmin/templates/cfs/Docs1011/CFS37/presentations/CFS37_Presentation_Global_RtF.pdf.

Dyck, Roland, Nathaniel Osgood, Tim Hsiang Lin, Amy Gao, and Mary Rose Stang. 2010. "Epidemiology of Diabetes Mellitus among First Nations and Non-First Nations Adults. *Canadian Medical Association Journal* 182 (3): 249–56.

Gignac, Julien. 2016. "Northern Ontario First Nations Declare Public-Health Emergency." *Globe and Mail*, 24 February.

Green, Chris, James F. Blanchard, T. Kue Young, and Jane Griffith. 2003. "The Epidemiology of Diabetes in the Manitoba-Registered First Nation People." *Diabetes Care* 26 (7): 1993–98.

Haman, François, Benedicte Fontaine-Bisson, Malek Batal, Pascal Imbeault, Jules M. Blais, and Michael A. Robidoux. 2010. "Obesity and Type 2 Diabetes in Northern Canada's Remote First Nations Communities: The Dietary Dilemma." *International Journal of Obesity* 34 (S2): S24–S31.

Hansen, Yolanda. 2011. "Growing Community: Community Gardens as a Local Practice of Food Sovereignty." In *Food Sovereignty in Canada: Creating Just and Sustainable Food Systems*, edited by Hannah Wittman, Annette Aurelie Desmarais, and Nettie Wiebe, 151–68. Winnipeg: Fernwood Publishing.

Imbeault, Pascal, François Haman, Jules M. Blais, Shinjini Pilon, Tim Seabert, Eva M. Krümmel, Michael A. Robidoux. 2011. "Obesity and Type 2 Diabetes Prevalence in Adults from Two Remote First Nations Communities in Northwestern Ontario, Canada." *Journal of Obesity* 2011: 1–5.

La Via Campesina. 2015. "International Peasant's Movement." Lia Via Campesina. https://viacampesina.org/en/index.php/organisation-mainmenu-44.

Mason, Courtney. 2014. *Spirits of the Rockies: Reasserting an Indigenous Presence in Banff National Park*. Toronto: University of Toronto Press.

McKay, Ian. 1994. *The Quest of the Folk: Antimodernism and Cultural Selection in Twentieth-Century Nova Scotia*. Montréal and Kingston: McGill-Queen's University Press.

Morrison, Dawn. 2008. *B.C. Food Systems Network Working Group on Indigenous Food Sovereignty: Final Activity Report*. Vancouver: BC Food Systems Network.

———. 2011. "Indigenous Food Sovereignty: A Model for Social Learning." In *Food Sovereignty in Canada: Creating Just and Sustainable Food Systems*, edited by Hannah Wittman, Annette Aurelie Desmarais, and Nettie Wiebe, 97–113. Winnipeg: Fernwood Publishing.

Popkin, Barry M., Bing Lu, and Fengying Zhai. 2002. "Understanding the Nutrition Transition: Measuring Rapid Dietary Changes in Transitional Countries." *Public Health Nutrition* 5 (6A): 947–53.

Power, Elaine M. 2011. "It's Time to Close Canada's Food Banks." *Globe and Mail*, 25 July.

Robidoux, Michael A., Pascal Imbeault, Jules M. Blais, Shinjini Pilon, Tim Seabert, Eva M. Krümmel, Malek Batal, A. Thériault, and François Haman. 2012. "Traditional Foodways in Two Contemporary Northern First Nations Communities." *Canadian Journal of Native Studies* 32 (1): 59–77.

Seabert, Tim, Shinjini Pilon, Bernard Pinet, François Haman, Pascal Imbeault, Michael A. Robidoux, Eva M. Krümmel, Linda E. Kimpe, and Jules M. Blais. 2014. "Elevated Contaminants Contrasted with Potential Benefits of Diversity of w-3 Fatty Acids in Wild Food Consumers of Two Remote First Nations Communities in Northern Ontario, Canada." *PLoS One* 9 (3): e90351, 1–10.

Snow, John. 2005. *These Mountains Are Our Sacred Places: The Story of the Stoney Indians*. Calgary: Fifth House Publishing.

Wiebe, Nettie, and Kevin Wipf. 2011. "Nurturing Food Sovereignty in Canada." In *Food Sovereignty in Canada: Creating Just and Sustainable Food Systems*, edited by Hannah Wittman, Annette Aurelie Desmarais, and Nettie Wiebe, 1–19. Winnipeg: Fernwood Publishing.

World Health Organization. 2015. http://www.who.int/en/.

Young, T. Kue, Jeff Reading, Brenda Elias, and John D. O'Neil. 2000. "Type 2 Diabetes Mellitus in Canada's First Nations: Status of an Epidemic in Progress." *Canadian Medical Association Journal* 163 (5): 561–66.

JOSEPH LEBLANC AND KRISTIN BURNETT

Chapter One

WHAT HAPPENED TO INDIGENOUS FOOD SOVEREIGNTY IN NORTHERN ONTARIO?

*Imposed Political, Economic,
Socio-Ecological, and Cultural Systems Changes*

Since the Second World War, governments, non-governmental organizations, the International Monetary Fund, and the World Bank have attempted to resolve hunger and malnutrition around the globe—a phenomenon commonly referred to as food insecurity—with solutions premised on increased economic growth and less market regulation. Such efforts are based on the assumption that poverty and inequity can be resolved through free-market capitalism and neoclassical economic thinking. At the World Health Summit of 1996, the World Health Organization (WHO) defined food security as existing "when all people at all times have access to sufficient, safe, nutritious food to maintain a healthy and active life" (World Health Organization 2015). The concept of food security has its limits and, according to William Schanbacher, reinforces a model that "reduces human relationships [with food] to their economic value" (2010, ix). Indeed, the concept of food security has systemically ensured that answers to hunger and malnourishment remain deeply rooted in economic and government-driven solutions where the power to initiate real change remains in the hands of a privileged few.

To date, efforts to address Indigenous food insecurity have been largely unsuccessful due to an ignorance of the historical factors that produced this food insecurity and the lack of initiative on the part of federal and provincial governments to undertake real systemic change. The Indigenous nations living in the geographic area that came to be known as Canada suffer from the cumulative impacts of many deliberate disruptions to their sovereignty. In this chapter, we hope to set the context for discussions of food insecurity in First Nations communities in Northern Ontario, by exploring significant historical disruptions to Indigenous food systems.

Where Are We Now?: Indigenous Food Security and Sovereignty

More conventional definitions of food security are tied to the ability of the individual or the household to purchase enough food to live an active, healthy life through participation in a market-based food system (Power 2008). In other words, people are reduced to consumers, and food insecurity, in this context, is regarded as primarily a symptom of poverty and inequality and not of larger factors rooted in a long history of colonialism and racism.[1] The failure of the food security framework to address the systemic imbalances that are entrenched in many political, social, and economic systems has led countless food activists to look for alternative models. Food sovereignty, a term coined at the Second International Assembly of La Via Campesina in Tlaxcala, Mexico, in 1996, has been increasingly employed because it acknowledges and names the "political and economic power dimensions inherent in the food and agricultural debate" (Wiebe and Wipf 2011, 3–4). Many different iterations of food sovereignty exist. For food activist Raj Patel, food sovereignty is a call to arms for those "who have systematically been excluded from the formulation of food policy, who have long been forced to live with the consequences of agrarian policy authored by those in cities with few, if any, links of accountability to those whose lives are wrecked by their ideas" (Patel n.d.). Other definitions emphasize the importance of cultural diversity, the values of mutual dependence, and an essential respect for the environment (see Schanbacher 2010; Windfuhr and Jonsen 2005; Amin 2011). One of the major goals of food sovereignty remains the desire to invert the structures of power and place the people who "produce, distribute, and consume food at the centre of decisions on food systems and policies" (Coxall 2014, 514).

However, even the above definitions are limiting because they fail to include the diversity of food systems, as well as the social meanings and relationships that different peoples and cultures have with their food and foodways, including those traditions that are central to the production and preparation of food. Definitions of food sovereignty need to go further than depicting human actions and concerns for the environment. They must embrace the value of and respect for the places where food is gathered and produced on cultural and spiritual levels while also addressing the power inequities and disconnections between the urban people who consume food and the rural/Indigenous people who harvest it. As Morrison has accurately pointed out, although Indigenous peoples did not originally use the language of food sovereignty, this concept was a "living reality" (Morrison 2011, 97) in Indigenous communities prior to contact and the introduction of Western economic practices and land management regimes, treaties, and residential schools. Currently, Indigenous peoples' systematic exclusion from the formulation of food policy occurs predominantly in the natural resource management sectors at the provincial level. They have long been forced to live with the consequences of extractive resource management planning undertaken by distant industries and policy makers.

Rural and remote northern Indigenous communities are currently experiencing disproportionate rates of household food insecurity. When combined with poverty, racism, historical and ongoing colonialism, and marginalization, this insecurity produces a multitude of health and social issues. In a 2004 federal government review of the food subsidy programs for northern communities, the study revealed that commercial food costs were 82 percent higher in Fort Severn, a Cree community located on Hudson Bay, than in Ottawa. In Fort Severn, the same review also revealed that two-thirds of the households were considered "food insecure" and at least one-quarter of the families had experienced hunger in the past twelve months because they were unable to afford food (Lawn and Harvey 2004). This was not a new situation for Fort Severn. Indian and Northern Affairs Canada (INAC) had undertaken a nutrition survey twelve years earlier and found that food insecurity had been a "serious concern" for the community's women: "approximately 45 percent of women in Fort Severn reported running out of money to buy food at least once a month in the past year, 39 percent reported not having enough to eat in the house in the past month, and about 40 percent of women were extremely concerned about not having enough money to buy food" (ibid., 1). More broadly, a 2008 Regional

Longitudinal Health Survey indicated that 17.8 percent of Indigenous adults age twenty-five to thirty-nine and 16.1 percent of Indigenous adults age forty to fifty-four in Canada reported going hungry due to lack of money in 2007–2008 (FNIGC 2012). While these statistics are extremely disturbing, they are nothing new. For Indigenous people in Canada, food insecurity is rooted in the history of the colonization of North America, beginning with the arrival of Europeans, the initiation of the fur trade, and the cumulative effects of government policy, residential schools, and race-based legislation that disadvantages Indigenous peoples.

Food insecurity of Indigenous peoples has become an invisible crisis in Canada—prevalent throughout hundreds of northern fly-in and rural communities but rarely visible to the urban masses, and thus to most Canadians. For the majority of Canadians, notions of food insecurity most often evoke images of starving children who live in faraway countries, their circumstances caused by catastrophic weather episodes, civil wars, and totalitarian regimes. Most Canadians do not envision obese Indigenous men, women, and children living on reserves in Northern Canada suffering from the effects of diabetes (Wiebe and Wipf 2011). Still, in Canada, Indigenous communities are attempting to rebuild the sovereignty that has been eroded over time due to the efforts of colonial governments and the Canadian state to destroy Indigenous food systems and a resilient way of life. Many individuals experience the consequences of food insecurity, which is expressed in high rates of diabetes, heart disease, and childhood obesity (National Aboriginal Health Organization 2012). Such ill health results from a lack of nutritious and affordable food choices, which is a by-product of the oligopolistic market food system (Patel 2007). In this system, a few large companies control all aspects of foods imported onto northern reserves, as well as the provision of food-producing resources such as seeds, traps, and nets. This form of external control was initiated under the federal government and extended through market monopolies and global capitalism. In contrast, food sovereignty is a political and social statement that calls for the right of people to define their own food systems or, in other words, to shape and craft food policy, but it does not fully incorporate beliefs that move beyond how food arrives at one's table. Also, food sovereignty is a limiting concept for many Indigenous peoples because it is premised on the transformation of a capitalist economic system that is already imposed. Making the existing system more egalitarian will not change the fundamental nature of the problem—the sustained imposition of alien economic and socio-cultural structures.

For Indigenous people, assessing food sovereignty must include matters that are not measurable according to Western concepts. Food sovereignty is not just about nutrition and affordability, but also about a connection to history, land/place, culture, and tradition. Anishinaabe food activist Winona LaDuke describes her people's connections to food: "for us, [food] comes from our relatives, whether they have wings or fins or roots, that is how we consider food. Food has a culture. It has a history. It has a story. It has relationships" (Platt 2013, para. 4). These interconnections are also deeply rooted in places where people have done things before, like blueberry picking or growing potatoes, and through the names people give these places (Norder 2012). The seemingly endless number of important places named "Potato Island," "Blueberry Hill," or "Moose River," across the North, offer intergenerational learning opportunities and reinforce positive, constructive behaviours of family and community building, in ways that the market food system never can.

Food insecurity and food sovereignty in Indigenous communities cannot be addressed without first understanding the challenges and transformations that Indigenous people have experienced and continue to endure since the arrival of Europeans in North America and the introduction of hierarchical economic, social, and political systems. The destruction of food economies that has led to food insecurity in Indigenous communities needs to be placed in its appropriate historical context in order for us to understand and address the ills of present-day realities. The spiritual oppression, produced by colonialism and food insecurity, is something that goes beyond food; even so, food remains a tangible way to begin the conversation about this injustice. Food is connected to all different systems, from the social and sacred to the economic and cultural. For Indigenous people, external control over their foodways and the erosion of their food sovereignty has been a central part of the colonial process. Below we briefly overview the transformative events that have shifted control over food processes and relationships from the local to the regional, national, and international.

Histories of Colonial Interference

Contact between Indigenous people and Europeans was not a single event, but rather the beginning of a series of ongoing encounters that continue to this day (Lutz 2007). During the early period of contact, trade sustained these encounters, creating new and different relationships between Indigenous peoples and Europeans. This led to the incorporation of Indigenous communities into a growing mercantilist, then capitalist, economy (see Ray 1974; Krech 1984). While Indigenous trade with Europeans was built upon existing trade networks that spread throughout the Americas, participating in Western economic systems was philosophically different from exchanges with other Indigenous nations. Trade for European goods brought Indigenous peoples into direct contact with Europeans and their world views.

Indigenous peoples were increasingly caught up in a growing web of production wherein, instead of producing and redistributing within local or regional systems, they became extractors and producers for much larger European markets (Innis 1999). While contact and the incorporation of Indigenous peoples in North America into the capitalist economy took place over a long period of time and in many different forms, perhaps one of the most damaging elements of this exchange was not material but philosophical. Often the incorporation of Indigenous peoples into European trading systems had immediate and visible effects; for instance, those Indigenous traders who adopted European ideologies of Christianity and/or capitalism accrued greater benefits. Initially, French traders restricted the exchange of guns to those Indigenous peoples who converted to Catholicism (Salisbury 1992), creating immediate and tangible rewards for participating Indigenous traders.

Increasing involvement in the fur trade also altered the political and social economy of Indigenous communities, as these "new modes of production favoured men over women, young over old, the individual over the group" (Klein 1983, 165). Trade and the accumulation of wealth changed the ways in which families and communities related to each other and introduced the idea that resources could go elsewhere and serve very little benefit to the community. The shift of resources from a closed system into an open one that did not embody similar world views regarding wealth and capital accumulation meant that there was little reciprocity in the exchange of goods. Instead, resources were drained from Indigenous communities

and their surrounding territories. The incorporation of Indigenous traders into a system premised upon the accumulation of individual wealth, to
further state and class interests, lay in direct contradiction to Indigenous
modes of community, reciprocity, mutual respect, and collective well-being.

In 1850, an Act for the Better Protection of the Lands and Property of
Indians in Lower Canada and an Act for the Protection of Indians in Upper
Canada from Imposition, and the Property Occupied or Enjoyed by them
from Trespass and Injury were passed. These acts were perhaps the most
significant pieces of legislation regarding Indigenous peoples in the geographic area that came to be known as Canada. The purpose of these acts
was to determine who belonged and who did not belong on this "protected"
land; to do so, the state needed to be able to define who was an Indian and
who was not. As a result, for the first time, Indigenous identity was codified
in law, without any consideration for existing self-determined membership
or community practices and relationships. Indians were defined as "all persons of Indian ancestry, and all persons married to such persons, belonging
to or recognized as belonging to an Indian band, and living with that band"
(Milloy 1991, 147). By creating a limited category or definition of "Indian"
the government ensured that Indigenous people and communities would
fight each other for access to dwindling resources.

To further erode Indigenous self-governance and control over their
lands, in 1857 Lower and Upper Canada passed an Act to Encourage the
Gradual Civilization of the Indian Tribes in this Province, and to Amend
the Laws Relating to Indians. It included the first enfranchisement provisions, whereby if Indigenous people met a particular set of criteria, they
could be stripped of their Indian status and be given the "privilege" of
becoming British citizens. Any Indian man over twenty-one who could
"speak, read, and write either English or in French language readily and
well, and [was] sufficiently advanced in the elementary branches of education and [was] of good moral character and free from debt" met these
criteria (Tobias 1983, 42–43).

Most significantly, the 1850 and 1857 acts led to the first national artic-
ulation of the characteristics and types of behaviours that came to represent
"civilized" actions for Indigenous populations (Tobias 1983). These legislative acts imposed a sweeping and universal definition of what it meant to

be an "Indian." The 1857 Act was followed by the 1869 Act for the Gradual Enfranchisement of Indians, the Better Management of Indian Affairs, and to Extend the Provisions of the Act 31st Victoria, which initiated a formal and concerted attack on Indigenous forms of governance by the Canadian state. This act imposed European-Canadian forms of governance, and ignored the fact that Indigenous nations had been self-governing since time immemorial. On reserves, the Crown reserved the right to remove from office those people considered unqualified or unfit to hold it. Usually it was those individuals who defied the Indian agent or refused to comply with the Department of Indian Affairs regulations (Miller 2000).

In 1876, all extant legislation pertaining to Indians was consolidated under the Indian Act. Over the next century, there were no fewer than fifty major amendments to the Indian Act, many of which were designed to further impose Euro-Canadian world views as well as modes of living, working, learning, and family life. Indeed, the 1884 and 1895 amendments, which criminalized the Sun Dance and Potlatch (and all giveaway ceremonies), were indicative of efforts to regulate economic behaviours and activities by prohibiting the redistribution of goods within communities. This resulted in the erosion of social cohesion, reciprocity, and well-being (see Pettipas 1994). In 1880, the federal government created a new branch in the civil service, the Department of Indian Affairs, in order to establish the formal means and necessary bureaucracy to manage Indians and lands reserved for Indians.

To solidify formal control over Indigenous peoples and their territories, the federal government was assigned exclusive jurisdiction over "Indians and all Indian land" under the 1867 British North America Act (now the Constitution Act) section 91, subsection 24 (Tobias 1983, 39). Besides creating a paternalistic system wherein Indigenous peoples would always be treated like children unable to manage their own affairs, sections 91 and 92 produced an ongoing jurisdictional nightmare in regards to the management of natural resources and to the delivery of key services. According to the British North America Act, all matters pertaining to "Indians" fall under federal authority. Whereas land management; health care (including prescription drug abuse clinics, annual food price monitoring, breastfeeding supports, etc.); infrastructure (such as roads, bridges, drinking water facilities, sewage, schools, airports, etc.); natural resources (including rivers and streams, exploration, hunting, trapping, resource development and extraction, silviculture, and watershed protection mechanisms such as conservation authorities); education; and child welfare all fall under provincial jurisdiction. As such, the provinces are not legally responsible for Indians or lands reserved for Indians, and various jurisdictions interpret their legal duties regarding Indigenous peoples very differently (Miller 2000).

In Ontario, the province has entered into service delivery agreements with the Government of Canada to provide social assistance. However, the Ontario Works program is applied universally throughout the province, without consideration for the varying rates of living expenses. The cost of living is significantly higher in many northern Indigenous communities compared to the rest of Ontario. Critics have called for the revision of social assistance mechanisms across Canada to amend inadequate funding for public health and food insecurity (De Schutter 2012). In urban centres, critics often base their recommendations on statistics generated through public health agencies and academic institutions; however, there are very few data service collection mechanisms for Indigenous peoples, especially those living on reserves. Therefore little data exists. Local boards of health in Southern Ontario have been collecting food prices annually using the Nutritious Food Basket program since 1974 (Ontario Ministry of Health 2010). In Northern Ontario, there is no such comprehensive, standardized monitoring of the cost of food. The only price "monitoring" mechanism that currently exists under Nutrition North Canada requires that certain food prices be self-reported by food vendors—in only sixteen of Ontario's 133 First Nations (Nutrition North Canada n.d.). As a result, foods marketed to on-reserve Indigenous peoples are virtually unregulated and the real cost of living is largely unknown. Without data to inform decision making, Indigenous issues are often relegated to a jurisdictional void without consistent funding, program access, or structural support.

In relation to land management, there exists a series of patchwork agreements negotiated between the federal and provincial governments with little input from Indigenous peoples. Moreover, what has become clear is that the different levels of government communicate very little with each other and, most often, the economic interests determine which policies and agreements are implemented or followed. This division of jurisdiction has led to conflict between provincial natural resource managers and the people who live on the land. For example, it is up to the provinces and their structures, in this case the ministry of Natural Resources, to decide if blueberries get sprayed in season with glyphosate[2]—even if Indigenous peoples are living in the region and harvesting food. As part of Ontario's forest management regimen, tens of thousands of hectares of young plantations or old harvested blocks are sprayed, with little regard for how the herbicide may affect the ways in which local people gather plants for food.

The Indian Act and the jurisdictional confusion that exists due to sections 91 and 92 of the British North America Act have relegated Indigenous peoples to a grey area in constitutional and legal matters. Many of the services and rights that are taken for granted by non-Indigenous people in Canada do not exist for on-reserve Indigenous peoples. Significantly, the Indian Act has restricted their ability to use and manage their lands as they had for generations. Indeed, the basis of all Indian legislation has been to force Indigenous people to adopt Euro-Canadian forms of governance, private property, individualism, and nuclear patriarchal families.

At the same time that the state began to pass legislation that would come to define identity and membership for many Indigenous peoples, the British Crown (in procedures later adopted and elaborated on by the federal government of Canada) also initiated the "modern" treaty-making process in the 1850s with the Robinson treaties (Robinson-Superior Treaty and Robinson-Huron Treaty) (Surtees 1986). William Robinson negotiated the Robinson Treaties primarily with the Ojibwa of the northern Great Lakes region. These early treaties established the template upon which the Canadian federal government would negotiate the numbered treaties. They all possess similar characteristics (with minor variations): the cession of land and creation of reserves, the guarantee of annuities, the description of the government's obligations and responsibilities, and the continued right to hunt and fish by Indians on Crown lands (Treaty 7 Elders and Tribal Council 1996). The treaty process then moved further west and then north to cover most of Canada except for British Columbia and the Arctic (see Long 2010; Switzer 2011; Miller 2009).

While there are vastly different interpretations and understandings of these treaties between the state and the different Indigenous groups who negotiated them, what is clear is that the treaties were used by the federal government to confine people to reserves. This compelled their transition from a mobile lifestyle, in which Indigenous people played an intimate role in the food system, to a sedentary lifestyle where people were increasingly reliant on commercial foods. The treaties involved giving up specific rights, which was not the intent of the people who signed them. According to Elders, treaties were meant to form the basis of a mutually beneficial relationship in which these lands were shared. Instead, the treaties gave Euro-Canadians a piece of paper, a justification to unilaterally build a country on ceded Indigenous lands without consideration for the peoples who had lived there since time immemorial.

The treaties confined Indigenous people to reserves, and until 1951 Indian agents were empowered to restrain their movements. For instance, people who wanted to leave their reserve or visit family on another reserve had to request permission from the Indian agent. In exercising these powers, government officials forced a transition to a static community model and prevented movement within the forest and freshwater food systems. The Indian agent also had the power to prevent people from hunting and fishing. No longer were communities able to make adjustments for environmental changes. When the flow of a river changed, for example, communities were unable to move to an area where they could access more resources. The federal government no longer allowed that kind of flexible and adaptable mobility, thus limiting the ability of Indigenous peoples to live in an interconnected relationship with nature.

In addition to directly undermining the ability of Indigenous communities to control and determine their own foodways in their territories, the federal government sought to ensure that the environmental and cultural knowledge would not be passed on from one generation to the next through the forcible transfer of children. Indeed, the removal of Indigenous children from their homes and communities by Euro-Canadians became a regular occurrence in Canada. The systematic internment of generations of children in Indian residential schools began in the 1870s and lasted until 1996 (see Chrisjohn and Young 1997; Milloy 1999; Miller 1996). As will be discussed in more depth in Chapter 4, most residential schools were harsh and violent institutions designed to assimilate children by severing their ties with family, community, and culture. In 1920, Duncan Campbell Scott, one of the major architects of Canadian Indian policy, described his mandate before a special parliamentary committee: "I want to get rid of the Indian problem. I do not think as a matter of fact, that this country ought to continuously protect a class of people who are unable to stand alone. That is my whole point. Our objective is to continue until there is not a single Indian in Canada that has not been absorbed into the body politic, and there is no Indian question, and no Indian Department" (Titley 1986, 50). In addition to the residential school system, after the Second World War, child welfare authorities seized thousands of Indigenous children under the guise of child protection. This era is infamously known as the "sixties scoop" (Sinclair 2007). In Northwestern Ontario from 1981 to 1982, Indigenous children made up 85 percent of the children in foster care (Mandell et al. 2003). The disproportionate representation of Indigenous children in the child welfare system persists to this day (Blackstock 2011).

The residential schools and the sixties scoop amounted to the systematic severing of the connections between parents and children. Parents were unable to teach their children place-based knowledge that they had learned from previous generations. Removed children were prevented from observing their relatives acting as self-sufficient and productive members of communities and they did not witness how people took care of each other. Children no longer learned the lesson that work and life-sustaining activities could and should be undertaken collectively for the good of the entire community.

The children were taught that their cultures were uncivilized and underdeveloped. They were forced into the Western world through Christianity, violence, and hard labour. For many survivors, their experiences in the schools included severe punishments that have left deep wounds. For example, the schools often used labour on their garden plots as punishment, and schoolchildren would be subjected to hours of intense labour, weeding, digging, and carrying water, for various infractions. Many were left with negative associations with that type of work; consequently, these individuals did not grow up to tend gardens, even though it was traditionally a common practice in Indigenous communities in this region. The removal of children and the use of food-procuring activities as forms of punishment undermined their sufficiency and served to sever the intergenerational transmission of ecological knowledge that could only be learned through observation and practice. As profiled in Chapter 5, communities are only now recovering from these broken intergenerational ties by reinvesting in land-based food programs for youth. Ultimately, residential schools disrupted community cohesion and compromised the values of mutual obligation and respect. The removal of children from their parents and communities had a deep and long-lasting legacy of violence and trauma.

Oligopolization of Imported Food, Fuel, and Supply Markets

An oligopolized market system exists throughout Northern Canada in regards to the provision of foods, fuel, and most general goods. This means that few actors with strong relationships control the various elements of this market-based system, including the supporting wholesale, distribution, transportation, retail, and banking industries. As a result, corporate interests have developed a sophisticated supply chain and support infrastructure. Indeed, the North West Company's Northern Stores, which hold approximately 50 percent of the market share in Northern Canada, reported record profits of $134.3 million in 2012 (CBC News 2013). Under this model, profit and growth dictate interchanges between people and the suppliers of their basic needs. Social accountability is only employed insofar as it is required by law. In an oligopolistic system, Indigenous food sovereignty is nearly impossible because the control of food economies lies in the hands of remote entities driven by profit margins.

As a result of the centralization of power and decision-making in the market-based food system, individuals are presented with few choices at high costs. Foods, fuel, clothing, toiletries, housewares, and even supplies supporting the participation in traditional food systems are offered through very few vendors. These vendors currently decide what is sold and at what price. As Chapter 2 demonstrates, prior to forced settlement on reserves, Indigenous peoples, in what is currently known as Northern Ontario, were permaculturalist hunter-gatherers with established local food systems. But the imposed changes significantly disrupted food production and distribution systems and endangered Indigenous food sovereignty. The global increase in consumption of highly processed, calorie-dense convenience and fast foods has also reached the remote forests of the North. In the 2000s, four Pizza Huts, five KFCs, and fourteen Fun 2 Go snack shops were opened on remote reserves in Northern Ontario, bringing greater access to convenience foods high in fats, salt, and refined carbohydrates. Therefore it is not a surprise that Indigenous peoples now comprise one of the unhealthiest segments of Ontario's population (Health Council of Canada 2005). Individuals with type 2 diabetes and heart disease are dependent on healthy diets for proper management of these chronic diseases; however, they are forced to continue to feed themselves from the same markets they always have. Healthy market foods are not offered for sale, or are of poor quality and thus unacceptable, or are prohibitively costly and therefore inaccessible.

The prevalence of diet-related diseases in Indigenous communities has supported the development of a significant health-promotion industry. Dietary patterns indicate a predominantly processed diet in Indigenous communities and the officials' response is to guide consumer choices within the existing market-based system (Chan et al. 2012). Unfortunately, it appears that these strategies are developed without a contextual understanding of how Indigenous food sovereignty has been eroded. The root cause of poor nutritional practices in Indigenous communities is not simply that people do not know what to eat. The reality is that nearly all aspects of Indigenous food systems have been disrupted, eroding Indigenous food sovereignty, health, and well-being.

Conclusion

Current food systems in Northern Ontario's Indigenous communities exist as a function of colonialism. If we were to draw an analogy between our[3] current food systems and a raging river, an observer standing on the river's edge sees our food systems as a permanent unmanageable force that moves without our involvement, and any efforts to alter the river's flow are swept away by its massive force. However, this river has not always been there and its energy once flowed elsewhere. Colonialism and its imposed disruptions not only changed the path of this flow of energy, it also redirected the river from the path that was carved over generations. While it would seem that, at this point, the easiest solution would be to jump into the river and be swept away, instead, we have learned that this energy does not lead to a good place, and that we must continue to place our stones in the river so that, over time and through our collective strength, we can change the current. We can disrupt the existing food system by not following the existing pathways and by creating new ones.

The solutions to food insecurity cannot emerge from within the existing dominant paradigm that has eroded Indigenous food sovereignty. The imposed disruptions to Indigenous food systems, discussed in this chapter, have had cumulative impacts greater than any single disruption. Indigenous people, traditions, and food systems are inherently resilient; however, the cumulative and multigenerational impacts of these changes have eroded our resiliency. This is not to say our independence cannot be restored, but the actors who operate the imposed Western food system hold Indigenous food sovereignty and well-being hostage. As we, Indigenous people, seek to rebuild food security and to return to a healthful life, we must reclaim our food sovereignty from external powers. Understanding how our food sovereignty was taken from us in the first place is a crucial step toward restoring our communities.

Notes

1. For more information about the most recent iteration of Canada's Food Guide, see Mahsa and L'Abbe (2015). For a discussion of the importance of considering the notion of cultural food security and Indigenous peoples, see Elaine Power (2008). She argues that food security conceptualizations, policies, and programs for Indigenous peoples need to consider both the market food system, but also traditional food systems.

2. Glyphosate is the world's most widely produced herbicide used to kill weeds. It was introduced by Monsanto in 1974 under the trade name Roundup. In March of 2015 the World Health Organization's International Agency for Research on Cancer classified glyphosate as "probably carcinogenic in humans." For more information see Cressey (2015) and Guyton and co-authors (2015).

3. Joseph LeBlanc is a member of the Odawa Nation and uses the broadly inclusive term "we" to refer to Indigenous nations/peoples generally.

References

Amin, Samin. 2011. "Food Sovereignty: A Struggle for Convergence in Diversity." Preface in *Food Movements Unite!: Strategies to Transform Our Food Systems*, edited by Eric Holt-Giménez, ix–xviii. Oakland, CA: Food First Books.

Blackstock, Cindy. 2011. "Wanted: Moral Courage in Canadian Child Welfare." *First Peoples Child and Family Review* 6 (2): 36–47.

CBC News. 2013. "North West Company Reports Record Profit," 25 April. http://www.cbc.ca/news/canada/north/north-west-company-reports-record-profit-1.1375327.

Chan, Laurie, Olivier Receveur, Donald Sharp, Harold Schwartz, Amy Ing, Karen Fediuk, Andrew Black, and Constantine Tikhonov. 2012. *First Nations Food, Nutrition and Environment Study (FNFNES): Results from Manitoba (2010).* Prince George, BC: University of Northern British Columbia.

Chrisjohn, Roland, and Sherri Young with Michael Maraun. 1997. *The Circle Game: Shadows and Substance in the Indian Residential School Experience in Canada.* Penticton, BC: Theytus Books.

Coxall, Malcom. 2014. *Ethical Eating: A Complete Guide to Sustainable Food.* Andalusia, Spain: Cornelia Books.

Cressey, Daniel. 2015. "Widely Used Herbicide Linked to Cancer." *Nature*, 24 March, http://www.nature.com/news/widely-used-herbicide-linked-to-cancer-1.17181.

De Schutter, Olivier. 2012. *Report of the Special Rapporteur on the Right to Food.* New York: United Nations General Assembly, Session 22. 24 December, 30–40.

FNIGC (First Nations Information Governance Centre). 2012. *First Nations Regional Longitudinal Health Survey (RHS) 2008/10: National Report on Adults, Youth and Children Living in First Nations Communities.* Ottawa: FNIGC. http://fnigc.ca/sites/default/files/docs/first_nations_regional_health_survey_rhs_2008-10_-_national_report.pdf.

Government of Canada. n.d. "Eligible Communities." Nutrition North Canada. http://www.nutritionnorthcanada.gc.ca/eng/1415540731169/1415540791407.

Guyton, Kathryn Z., Dana Loomis, Yann Grosse, Fatiha El Ghissassi, Lamia Benbrahim-Tallaa, Neela Guha, Chiara Scoccianti, Heidi Mattock, and Kurt Straif. 2015. "Carcinogenicity of Tetrachlorvinphos, Parathion, Malathion, Diazinon, and Glyphosate." *Lancet* 16 (5): 490–91.

Health Council of Canada. 2005. *The Health Status of Canada's First Nations, Metis, and Inuit Peoples.* Toronto: Health Council of Canada. http://publications.gc.ca/collections/collection_2012/ccs-hcc/H174-37-2005-1-eng.pdf.

Indian and Northern Affairs Canada. 2010. *A History of Treaty-Making in Canada.* Gatineau, QC: Indian and Northern Affairs Canada.

Innis, Harold A. 1999. *The Fur Trade in Canada: An Introduction to Canadian Economic History.* 2nd. ed. Toronto: University of Toronto Press.

Klein, Alan. 1983. "The Political-Economy of Gender: A 19th Century Plains Indian Case Study." In *The Hidden Half: Studies of Plains Indian Women*, edited by Patricia Albers and Beatrice Medicine, 143–74. Lanham, MD: University Press of America.

Krech III, Shepard. 1984. *The Subarctic Fur Trade: Native Social and Economic Adaptations.* Vancouver: UBC Press.

Lawn, Judith, and Dan Harvey. 2004. *Nutrition and Food Security in Fort*

Severn, Ontario: Baseline Survey for the Food Mail Pilot Project. Ottawa: Indian and Northern Affairs Canada.

Long, John S. 2010. *Treaty No. 9: Making the Agreement to Share the Land in Far Northern Ontario in 1905.* Montreal: McGill-Queen's University Press.

Lutz, John Sutton. 2007. "First Contact as a Spiritual Performance: Encounters on the North American West Coast." In *Myth and Memory: Stories of Indigenous-European Contact,* edited by John Sutton Lutz, 30–45. Vancouver: UBC Press.

Mahsa, J. and M. L'Abbe. 2015. "The Time for an Updated Canadian Food Guide Has Arrived." *Applied Physiology, Nutrition, and Metabolism* 40 (8): 854–57.

Mandell, Deena, Joyce Clouston Carlson, Marshall Fine, and Cindy Blackstock. 2003. *Aboriginal Child Welfare: Partnerships for Children and Families Project.* Waterloo, ON: Wilfrid Laurier University.

Martin, Debbie. 2012. "Nutrition Transition and the Public-Health Crisis: Aboriginal Perspectives on Food and Eating." In *Critical Perspectives in Food Studies,* edited by Mustafa Koç, Jennifer Sumner, and Anthony Winson, 208–22. Don Mills: Oxford University Press.

Miller, J. R. 1996. *Shingwauk's Vision: A History of Native Residential Schools.* Toronto: University of Toronto Press.

——. 2000. *Skyscrapers Hide the Heavens: A History of Indian-White Relations in Canada.* 3rd edition. Toronto: University of Toronto Press.

——. 2009. *Compact, Contract, Covenant: Aboriginal Treaty-Making in Canada.* Toronto: University of Toronto Press.

Milloy, John S. 1991. "The Early Indian Acts: Developmental Strategy and Constitutional Change." In *Sweet Promises: A Reader on Indian-White Relations in Canada,* edited by J. R.

Miller, 145–54. Toronto: University of Toronto.

——. 1999. *A National Crime: The Canadian Government and the Residential School System, 1879 to 1986.* Winnipeg: University of Manitoba Press.

Morrison, Dawn. 2011. "Indigenous Food Sovereignty: A Model for Social Learning." In *Food Sovereignty in Canada: Creating Just and Sustainable Food Systems,* edited by Hannah Wittman, Annette Aurelie Desmarais, and Nettie Wiebe, 97–113. Winnipeg: Fernwood Publishing.

National Aboriginal Health Organization. 2012. *Aboriginal Children and Obesity,* Fact Sheet. http://www.naho.ca/documents/naho/english/factSheets/2012_05_childhood_obesity.pdf.

Norder, John. 2012. "The Creation and Endurance of Memory and Place among First Nations of Northwestern Ontario, Canada." *International Journal of Historical Archaeology* 16 (2): 385–400.

Ontario Ministry of Health. 2010. *Nutritious Food Basket: Guidance Document.* Queen's Printer for Ontario.

Patel, Raj. n.d. "Food Sovereignty: A Brief Introduction." Personal Website. http://rajpatel.org/2009/11/02/food-sovereignty-a-brief-introduction/.

——. 2009. *Stuffed and Starved: The Hidden Battle for the World's Food System.* Toronto: Harper Perennial.

Pettipas, Katherine. 1994. *Severing the Ties that Bind: Government Repression of Indigenous Religious Ceremonies on the Prairies.* Winnipeg: University of Manitoba Press.

Platt, John. 2013. "Why Winona LaDuke is Fighting for Food Sovereignty." *Mother Nature Network,* 4 March. http://www.mnn.com/leaderboard/stories/why-winona-laduke-is-fighting-for-food-sovereignty.

Power, Elaine M. 2008. "Conceptualizing Food Security for Aboriginal People in Canada." *Canadian Journal of Public Health* 99 (2): 95–97.

Ray, Arthur J. 1974. *Indians in the Fur Trade: Their Role as Trappers, Hunters, and Middlemen in the Lands Southwest of the Hudson's Bay, 1660–1870.* Toronto: University of Toronto Press.

Salisbury, Neal. 1992. "Religious Encounters in a Colonial Context: New England and New France in the Seventeenth Century." *American Indian Quarterly* 16 (4): 501–9.

Schanbacher, William D. 2010. *The Politics of Food: The Global Conflict between Food Security and Food Sovereignty.* Santa Barbara, CA: Praeger.

Sinclair, Raven. 2007. "Identity Lost and Found: Lessons from the Sixties Scoop." *First Peoples Child and Family Review* 3 (1): 65–82.

Surtees, Robert J. 1986. *Treaty Research Report: The Robinson Treaties (1850).* Ottawa: Treaties and Historical Research Centre, Indian and Northern Affairs Canada.

Switzer, Maurice. 2011. *We Are All . . . Treaty People.* North Bay, ON: Union of Ontario Indians.

Titley, E. Brian. 1986. *A Narrow Vision: Duncan Campbell Scott and the Administration of Indian Affairs in Canada.* Vancouver: University of British Columbia Press.

Tobias, John L. 1983. "Protection, Civilization, Assimilation: An Outline History of Canada's Indian Policy." In *As Long as the Sun Shines and Water Flows: A Reader in Canadian Native Studies,* edited by Ian A.L. Getty and Antoine S. Lussier, 39–55. Vancouver: UBC Press.

Treaty 7 Elders and Tribal Council with Walter Hildebrandt, Dorothy First Rider, and Sarah Carter. 1996. *The True Spirit and Original Intent of Treaty 7.* Montreal: McGill-Queen's University Press.

Wiebe, Nettie, and Kevin Wipf. 2011. "Nurturing Food Sovereignty in Canada." In *Food Sovereignty in Canada: Creating Just and Sustainable Food Systems,* edited by Hannah Wittman, Annette Aurelie Desmarais, and Nettie Wiebe, 1–19. Winnipeg: Fernwood Publishing.

Windfuhr, Michael, and Jennie Jonsen. 2005. *Food Sovereignty: Towards Democracy in Localized Food Systems.* Rugby, Warwickshire, UK: ITDG Publishing.

World Health Organization. 2015. "Food Security." World Health Organization. http://www.who.int/foodsafety/areas_work/nutrition/en/.

FRANÇOIS HAMAN, BÉNÉDICTE FONTAINE-BISSON,
SHINJINI PILON, BENOÎT LAMARCHE, AND MICHAEL A. ROBIDOUX

Chapter Two

UNDERSTANDING THE LEGACY OF COLONIAL CONTACT FROM A PHYSIOLOGICAL PERSPECTIVE

*Nutrition Transitions and the Rise of Dietary
Disease in Northern Indigenous Peoples*

As eloquently described in Chapter 1, Indigenous peoples of Canada had an intimate understanding of food ecosystem dynamics, which enabled efficient harvesting of local food sources with optimal rates of success. In the region of Northwestern Ontario, specifically, people needed to be energy efficient to survive in an often harsh and unforgiving environment. As alluded to in the introduction, this ecological knowledge about living on the land was developed over thousands of years. Teachings were transferred from generation to generation to support community efforts to survive and thrive on the land. However, European contact and the various colonial practices significantly impacted Indigenous food systems. Over a short period of time, Indigenous peoples in this region went from a semi-nomadic lifestyle, relying entirely on off-the-land foods, to a more sedentary existence, with a strong dependency on processed Western foods (Bishop 1970; Ray 1998). Under these conditions, the incidence of diet-related chronic diseases, such as obesity and type 2 diabetes, quickly surpassed rates found in any non-Indigenous Canadian populations (Haman et al. 2010). In the province of Ontario, Ojibwa, Oji-Cree, and Cree communities have undergone tremendous lifestyle transformations despite their rural, remote, and northern locations. One consequence of these transformations is the alarming increase in the rates of obesity and obesity-related diseases (de-Gonzague et al. 1999; Gittelsohn et al. 1998; Szathmáry, Ritenbaugh, and

Goodby 1987; Young et al. 2000), which are some of the highest in the world (Harris et al. 1997; Seabert et al. 2013).

Over the past thirty years, researchers have attempted to identify biological explanations for the higher than normal increase in obesity and type 2 diabetes in children and adults living in isolated Indigenous communities. Various arguments have been put forward attempting to link the high prevalence of obesity-related diseases to some genetic deficiency that makes Indigenous peoples ill-equipped to contend with contemporary Western diets and living conditions. The message that accompanies these explanations not only underemphasizes the many complexities of health in Indigenous communities and the multipronged approaches required to address these challenges, it also serves to pathologize Indigenous peoples as fatalistically determined to become obese and to develop some type of chronic disease. In the following chapter we first consider the physiological impacts of the abrupt changes faced by Indigenous peoples, changes resulting from the disruption of local food systems, and the compromised nutrition in many northern communities (as outlined in Chapter 1). Second, we briefly tackle scientific research that explores the potential presence of genetic predispositions in Indigenous populations. These predispositions supposedly promote metabolic intolerance to the increased Westernization of dietary and lifestyle practices. By addressing the limitations and flaws in genetic determinism, we dismiss the perceived inevitability of the onset of chronic disease and provide practical and manageable solutions to the gross health disparities Indigenous peoples encounter (as discussed in Chapters 3, 4, and 5). For example, even minimal changes, such as an attempt to alter dietary intake, can lead to significant improvement in people's lives. The challenge then becomes how to increase food access and provide the means by which northern residents can get regular access to nutritious food.

The Great Disruption: From Self-Reliance to Dependency on Westernized Foods

Prior to European contact, for sustenance Indigenous peoples of Canada relied on the land or the sea, which comprised a wide variety of animal and plant species. Dietary practices were regionally and historically diverse. Some Indigenous groups drew almost entirely on animal food sources, while others benefited more significantly from agriculturally produced foods (Kuhnlein, Soueida, and Receveur 1996; Kwon et al. 2007). In Northern Canada, historical diets would have involved eating all food sources available on the land at any particular time, and consuming almost all parts of the animals (including liver, gonads, gut, brain, and bone marrow) (Robidoux, Haman, and Sethna 2009). These diets were considered mostly carnivorous and provide low amounts of carbohydrates (or sugars) and large quantities of animal lipids (or fats) and proteins. Carbohydrates were obtained only seasonally from wild plants and berries. In contrast to more contemporary diets, such a diet would have contained no refined sugars and would have been lower in industrially produced trans fat, but rich in vital nutrients, such as essential fatty acids, vitamins, and minerals (Appavoo, Kubow, and Kuhnlein 1991; Wein 1995; Receveur, Boulay, and Kuhnlein 1997; Belinsky and Kuhnlein 2000; Blanchet et al. 2000; Das 2000; Kuhnlein et al. 2002; Nakano et al. 2005a; Kuhnlein and Receveur 2007). Even though the types of local food recently consumed have been well-studied in various regions of Canada (Appavoo, Kubow, and Kuhnlein 1991; Wein 1995; Kuhnlein, Soueida, and Receveur 1996; Campbell et al. 1997; Gittelsohn et al. 1998; deGonzague et al. 1999; Belinsky and Kuhnlein 2000; Blanchet et al. 2000; Kuhnlein 2004; Batal et al. 2005; Nakano et al. 2005b; Kuhnlein and Receveur 2007; Berti, Soueida, and Kuhnlein 2008; Kuhnlein et al. 2008), the exact proportions of macronutrients and micronutrients traditionally consumed in an exclusively off-the-land diet remain difficult to assess. Historical accounts seldom specify proportions of various species and the parts of animal tissue consumed. Variations in total local food intake were greatly linked to seasonal availability of foods and to preparation practices. In any event, it is clear that fats were particularly valued as energy-dense nutrients, essential to sustain the physical demands of hunting, fishing, gathering, and domestic activities (Robidoux et al. 2009).

Sustaining these traditional food practices was extremely challenging as they required substantial harvesting efforts, planning, and perseverance. Prior to European contact, Indigenous peoples lived semi-nomadically in small groups following local food sources (Bishop 1984). Food practices that extracted the maximum amount of nutrients from gathered foods were essential to ensure that energy requirements were met. These food practices persisted well into the mid-1900s. As an example, a woman from the Sandy Lake First Nation, in Northwestern Ontario, recalled the exhaustive use of moose meat in her diet in the 1950s:

> We would take everything, even the inside of the moose,
> the stomach area and everything, you eat it. Even the nails
> [hooves] and underneath, that's the marrow, moose marrow
> from the bones, you don't throw anything away. The fat from
> the moose, you cut it up and you fry it—the inside from the
> moose, the fat, there's lots of fat there. You take that off and
> you put it into a pan outside where you make a fire, you put
> it into the pan and you fry it, and there's lots of grease and oil
> that comes from the fat. And that's how you make the moose
> fat. And you keep that as it kind of gets hard after a while.
> (Robidoux et al. 2009, 18)

Because animal and plant availability varied greatly, seasonally and regionally, food preservation was particularly important to sustain energy demands throughout the year. Smoking meats reduced its water content and created a protective coating from the wood oils. Plants and fruits could be dried. The harvested fats could be mixed with the preserved meat protein and dried berries.

In Indigenous communities of Northwestern Ontario, permanent settlements were established in the latter half of the twentieth century, as a result of Treaty 9 and its adhesions in the 1930s. This instituted a progressive reliance on store-bought foods and a decrease in land-based diets (Szathmáry, Ritenbaugh and Goodby 1987; Young 1994). In some communities, access to store-bought processed foods increased significantly over a fifty-year period. The changes in physical activity patterns, along with the presence of permanent stores and readily available lower-quality market food options, led to an excess in energy intake. This excess included the consumption of large quantities of processed fats, including industrially produced trans fat, refined sugars, and salt in the form of snack foods and soft drinks. Not only did access to these highly processed, highly palatable foods increase energy intake beyond daily requirements, it had an important effect on the manner in which wild food was being harvested, processed, and consumed. The consumption of off-the-land foods involved eating whatever was available at any particular time, and in all cases, almost all parts of the food sources were consumed.

In a study conducted by Robidoux, Haman, and Sethna (2009), Elders from the Sandy Lake First Nation, aged between sixty-five and eighty-two, were asked to recall life before the permanent presence of the Hudson's Bay store (later renamed the Northern Store) in the 1940s. While the locals did trade for flour, sugar, and tea at the Hudson's Bay store on the north shore of Big Sandy Lake, survival was based primarily on food acquired through hunting, fishing, and gathering. Elders were interviewed about the types of land-based food sources they consumed growing up in the region. One woman identified muskrats and squirrels as important food sources: "We would smoke it [the muskrat] and that's how we would prepare it . . . in the spring when all the squirrels were running about, my father would go around and collect all the squirrels and put them in the oven" (Robidoux, Haman, and Sethna 2009, 18). Another woman responded more generally, by saying, "Whatever we killed, that's what we ate" (ibid.). While this approach to off-the-land food consumption is still practised by some people, most rely on store-bought foods and have lost important ties to off-the-land-food practices. Reasons for these changes are multi-faceted—the depletion of wild food sources as a result of the fur trade; treaty-imposed settlement patterns and the introduction of permanent stores; the residential school system, which disrupted the intergenerational transmission of land-based skills; and the degradation of Indigenous culture as a result of colonialism—but it is widely believed that these lifestyle transitions are largely responsible for the significant rise in rates of obesity and obesity-related diseases in this region. These include: type 2 diabetes (Bruce 2000; Young et al. 2000; Johnson, Martin, and Sarin 2002), hypertension (Hegele et al. 1997), dyslipidemia (Daniel et al. 2001), and cardiovascular diseases (CVD) (Anand et al. 2001).

As a result of these dietary challenges, Indigenous peoples in Northwestern Ontario are facing some of the highest rates of diet-related diseases in the world. Several studies have documented the increasing levels of overweight and obesity in Canadians (Katzmarzyk 2002; Tremblay,

Katzmarzyk, and Willms 2002; Tjepkema 2006). The most recent data indicates that obesity (defined as a body mass index over 30 kg/m$^{2)}$ has increased from 14 percent in 1978/79 to 23 percent in 2004 among Canadian adults (Tjepkema 2006). The results from the 2004 Canadian Community Health Survey show that the prevalence of obesity is at 38 percent among Canadian Indigenous populations (living off reserve), bestowing this group with the highest prevalence of obesity in Canada (Katzmarzyk 2008).

In 2007, to better understand the impact of these dietary transitions on Indigenous peoples living in Northwestern Ontario, our Indigenous Health Research Group conducted studies in Kasabonika Lake First Nation and Wapekeka First Nation, documenting dietary practices and various health parameters. These two Northwestern Ontario, Oji-Cree First Nations are remote fly-in communities located approximately 615 kilometres north of Thunder Bay. There are approximately 300 people living in Wapekeka and 800 people living in Kasabonika Lake. Like other Indigenous communities in this region, they are accessible year-round by air and during the coldest winter months by a winter road constructed over snow and ice, allowing for the transportation of major supplies such as fuel and construction materials. In these communities, the typical diet is composed of both traditional and store-bought foods, in varying proportions (Robidoux et al. 2012). Traditional dietary practices persist despite tremendous efforts and costs associated with maintaining these practices. Still, local food access is limited, in a region desperately needing adequate nutrition, and valuable connections between land and people are weakened. In this study, our research focussed on establishing whether off-the-land food practices could provide sufficient amounts of nutritious wild food to reduce the prevalence of obesity and type 2 diabetes.

To achieve our objective, we first quantified the consumption of off-the-land foods using a mixed-research approach, combining formal interviews, dietary questionnaires, and biomarker techniques (e.g., profiling of stable isotopes and fatty acids found in the foods consumed) (Seabert et al. 2013). Through this work, we found significant differences in the amounts of wild food consumed among community members. At the extremes, some participants consumed wild food at least twice a week, while others ate it less than once a month. Even though this difference in the consumption of nutritious foods showed great promise in terms of dealing with chronic diseases, it did not show that this higher reliance on wild food could reduce rates of obesity and type 2 diabetes. In fact, the prevalence of overweight and obesity was comparable between the high wild-food group and the low wild-food group, with both averaging close to 96 percent (Imbeault et al. 2012). To compare levels of type 2 diabetes between high wild-food eaters versus low wild-food eaters, differences in insulin sensitivity were assessed by measuring glucose levels in a fasting state through a glucose tolerance test (ingestion of seventy-five grams of glucose to evaluate the evolution of glucose and insulin blood levels over two hours). Our results indicated that changes in blood glucose concentrations were not different between high wild-food eaters and low wild-food eaters. Of the seventy-two participants, twenty-six (36 percent) were considered diabetic based on the World Health Organization reference points. In addition, waist circumferences were measured to evaluate the regional accumulation of body fat at the abdominal level. Within the last decade, clinical researchers have established that an excess accumulation of body fat, namely at the abdominal level, is associated with a cluster of metabolic abnormalities often referred to as the metabolic syndrome (Eckel, Grundy, and Zimmet 2005; Després et al. 2008).

These results are not only alarming, but they highlight the extent to which poor nutrition can impact physiological health. In these communities, results related to rates of overweight (33 percent) and obesity (66 percent), type 2 diabetes (36 percent) and waist circumference (115 cm), exceeded all previously reported prevalence values. For example, the 2002–2003 First Nations Regional Longitudinal Health Survey collected data from on-reserve First Nations populations and showed that the self-reported prevalence of obesity was 31 percent (Committee 2005). This rate was 35 percent lower than the recorded level of obesity in the sample from the two Northern Ontario Oji-Cree communities. Of great concern also is the prevalence of type 2 diabetes measuring at 36 percent for the two participating communities, which is approximately six times higher than that found amongst non-Indigenous peoples in Canada. Waist circumference was also used to determine increased risks of developing diseases such as type 2 diabetes, hypertension, and atherosclerosis. Based on the Canadian guidelines for body-weight classification in adults, a waist circumference over or equal to 102 centimetres in men and 88 centimetres in women has been associated with a high risk for developing chronic diseases. We found that thirty-nine of the forty-one women, and twenty-six out of the thirty-one men who participated in this study showed values associated with increased health risks. The question remains, why is the prevalence of obesity and obesity-related diseases so high in this region? For some researchers, the explanation lies in genetics and in the controversial and persistent notion that Indigenous peoples from this region carry genetic variations that lead to increased prevalence of obesity-related chronic diseases.

Gene-Diet Interactions among Indigenous Peoples

There is little doubt that genes inherited from our ancestors play a role in determining our appearance, anatomy, and metabolic functioning. However, understanding how this genetic makeup and our environment interact to prevent or trigger disease development is far more difficult. Diet is a major environmental factor which interacts with the genome, an organism's DNA, to influence all bodily functions involved in health maintenance or disease development (Gillies 2003; Ordovas and Mooser 2004). Nutrients (carbohydrates, fats, proteins, vitamins, and minerals) and other food compounds can regulate the process by which genes are utilized by cells in the body (Simopoulos 2010). As these nutrients interact with the body, genes are critical for enabling blood sugar to enter cells (through insulin), for food to be digested (through enzymes), for blood to clot (through coagulation factors), and for tissues to be developed (Weiss and Tackney 2012). Nutrients do not only impact the way genes are being used to make proteins, but genetic variations also alter the way individuals respond to those same nutrients (Gillies 2003; Ordovas and Mooser 2004). Clearly, diet through its impact on gene expression and protein functions will affect health maintenance or disease development. In view of the markedly higher prevalence of chronic diseases in Indigenous Canadian populations, the question that is repeatedly asked is: are Indigenous peoples genetically ill-equipped to manage the highly processed and energy-dense diets of contemporary Western society?

A number of studies have attempted to quantify the relationship between the presence of certain gene variants and diet-related chronic diseases in Oji-Cree peoples of Northwestern Ontario. Conclusions from this work clearly emphasize that genetic makeup alone cannot explain the high rates of obesity and obesity-related diseases in these communities. Researchers focussed on specific gene variants generally associated with high rates of obesity, type 2 diabetes, and cardiovascular disease. These included variants of the peroxisome proliferator-activated receptor-g2 gene (PPAR-g2), the fatty acid-binding protein-2 gene (FABP2), and the common genetic variant in the obesity gene (FTO). While some of these gene variants are present within Oji-Cree peoples, researchers agree that they alone cannot be responsible for the high rates of dietary chronic diseases (Hegele et al. 2000). For example, the presence of the PPAR-g2, FABP2, and FTO gene variations was confirmed in one Oji-Cree community and associated with an increased risk of developing obesity, type 2 diabetes, and cardiovascular disease (Hegele et al. 2000; Hegele et al. 1996; Hegele et al. 1997). However, when the same variants were found in non-Indigenous populations, they provided a protective effect against these chronic diseases, possibly due to other differences in the genetic background or environmental factors (Deeb et al. 1998; Lear et al. 2011). In another study in the Sandy Lake First Nation (Ley et al. 2011), it was discovered that carriers of a genetic variant (hepatic nuclear factor-1a gene) had close to a four-fold increased risk of developing type 2 diabetes, yet active smokers carrying this gene variation were seven times more likely to develop type 2 diabetes. What this suggests is that, in this cohort, smoking was likely a greater contributing factor to the development of type 2 diabetes than genetic variation alone.

If one also takes into consideration the percentage of body fat, triglycerides (fat in the blood), and an elevated waist circumference, there is an even greater risk of developing chronic diseases. For example, individuals from this same community who were carriers of a specific genetic variation and who also had a combination of high triglycerides and elevated waist circumference were five times more likely to develop type 2 diabetes compared to those with low triglycerides and lower waist circumference (Pollex et al. 2006). Finally, another study (Hegele 1999) suggested that Oji-Cree peoples in Northwestern Ontario, and Inuit from the Keewatin region of Nunavut, have a higher prevalence of genetic variations which predispose them to type 2 diabetes and coronary heart disease. Based on this perceived genetic disposition, it would seem safe to assume that both Indigenous groups would have a higher risk of developing these diseases. However, the prevalence of diabetes and coronary heart disease is much lower among Inuit peoples, in contrast to Oji-Cree peoples (ibid.). These studies suggest that when looking for answers about the potential relationship between genetic makeup and the development of dietary diseases, risks of these diseases must be considered within the broad array of environmental and lifestyle factors.

In the examples above, researchers are attempting to understand how genetic disposition can increase risks of developing chronic diseases in some individuals (or groups) and have a protective effect in others, depending on key physiological markers of disease (e.g., waist circumference, high blood fat, obesity) and environmental factors (e.g., physical activity, smoking). What is evident from these studies is that genetic variations on their own cannot explain the significant rise in obesity and obesity-related diseases in some Indigenous communities. Inherited susceptibility to disease depends, to a large extent, on an individual's environmental exposure, diet, and lifestyle. While genetic drift (change in genetic variation frequency in a population due to random mating) takes multiple generations to occur, the environment can change more rapidly and drastically (Jobling 2012). In addition, each individual genetic variation plays a minor role in disease development, compared to the complex array of health determinants impacting the diet-related chronic diseases in Indigenous groups. The sudden shift from land-based food practices has led to an increase in the consumption of highly refined, calorie-dense foods, and a decrease in physical activity. Compounding these significant lifestyle and dietary changes are the exorbitant costs of market foods. Considering the high levels of unemployment in most northern communities, it is almost impossible for residents to afford regular access to nutritious foods. While research focussing on the genetic implications of chronic disease development is theoretically interesting, it is of little consequence when considering the myriad factors contributing to the disproportionately high burden of diet-related chronic diseases in Indigenous communities. Instead, the focus must shift to dietary intake, and the many challenges remote rural Indigenous communities face to get access to nutritious foods and to make optimal decisions about consuming them.

Feeding the North to Reduce Diet-Related Chronic Diseases
There is a wealth of scientific data indicating that a large proportion of chronic diseases can be prevented early in life through healthier lifestyles, including healthier dietary behaviour. This is particularly true during pregnancy and infancy, where diet has profound effects on short- and long-term health (Solomons 2009). The environmental exposure in utero and early life, two critically sensitive windows of development, can permanently alter the genome and increase susceptibility to chronic diseases later in life (Vanhees et al. 2014). Maternal malnutrition and suboptimal intrauterine environment—gestational diabetes, obesity, exposure to contaminants, usage of alcohol, drugs, or smoking—induce adaptive metabolic and physiologic changes in the foetus, by permanently altering the structure of the genome (the study of these adaptations is called epigenetics). These changes can result in abnormal functioning of cells, organs, and tissues, leading to an increased risk of developing chronic diseases in adulthood. A growing number of animal and epidemiological studies in humans have revealed that inadequate nutrition during pregnancy is associated with heightened risk of obesity, type 2 diabetes, cardiovascular diseases, and cancer. Diet during infancy, which includes breastfeeding, as well as diet during childhood, and a choice of complementary foods and dietary patterns also have a crucial impact on short- and long-term health. Clearly, the foods we have access to and the amounts we eat at all stages of the life cycle have a tremendous impact on our overall health and susceptibility to diseases.

Unfortunately, many Indigenous communities in Northern Canada have limited access to nutritious foods, in large part due to high costs of shipping goods to these remote regions (Chan et al. 2006; Lambden et al. 2006). The exorbitant costs of market foods throughout the North have led to recent calls for a resurgence in local modes of food procurement—which in northern Indigenous communities primarily involve hunting, fishing, and gathering. A 2009 report on the Canadian Arctic (INAC 2009) cited land-based foods as a nutritious, cheaper, and more culturally relevant option in combatting issues of food insecurity for northern Indigenous peoples. While there are important benefits to northern land-based diets, research conducted by our group points to the critical barriers that many communities face in acquiring sufficient amounts of wild food for regular consumption, despite the relative abundance of wild food sources in most northern regions (Pal, Haman, and Robidoux 2013). In part due to the loss of intergenerational sustenance-related knowledge and skills, such as tracking animals, setting nets for fish, and land-based survival skills, individuals and groups in many Indigenous communities are struggling to harvest land-based foods and also have little access to healthy, quality market foods. Communities are still searching for solutions to this contemporary dietary dilemma.

Conclusion

There is now little doubt that Indigenous peoples of Northern Canada have undergone profound changes in dietary habits and lifestyle behaviours, which have led to a significant rise in obesity and obesity-related diseases. In this context, research agrees that genetic variations and predispositions do not alone explain this alarmingly high prevalence in diet-related chronic diseases. The inherited susceptibility to disease depends to a large extent on individual environmental exposure, diet, and lifestyle. We can establish more adequate and effective dietary strategies to address northern food security and the high prevalence of diet-related diseases by moving beyond genetic explanations and the further stigmatization of Indigenous peoples as fatalistically determined to become obese and to develop obesity-related diseases. While several organizations have developed healthy-eating guidelines and messages, these remain unsuccessful, impractical, and ill-adapted to the nutritional issues faced in the North and specifically in Indigenous communities. With healthy food options being too expensive and limited, low-quality, store-bought foods generally become the most affordable and easily available alternatives. Re-introducing off-the-land food strategies in a community context must be weighed against the variations in land use or access, health of the people, local knowledge competencies, and environmental conditions, including levels of environmental contaminants. In this context, community-based food initiatives are essential to orchestrate practical strategies aimed at dealing with issues of malnutrition and chronic disease. Researchers agree that there is a sense of urgency as the ill effects of improper diet are becoming more and more apparent in children and youth. We need to make fundamental changes and take immediate action if solutions to these major health problems in northern Indigenous communities are to be reached.

References

Anand, Sonia S., Salim Yusuf, R. Jacobs, A.D. Davis, Qilong Yi, H. Gerstein, P.A. Montague, and Eva Lonn. 2001. "Risk Factors, Atherosclerosis, and Cardiovascular Disease among Aboriginal People in Canada: The Study of Health Assessment and Risk Evaluation in Aboriginal Peoples (SHARE-AP)." *Lancet* 358 (9288): 1147–53.

Appavoo, Donna M., Stan Kubow, and Harriet V. Kuhnlein. 1991. "Lipid Composition of Indigenous Foods Eaten by the Suhtú (Hareskin) Dene-Métis of the Northwest Territories." *Journal of Food Composition and Analysis* 4 (2): 107–19.

Batal, Malek, Katherine Gray-Donald, Harriet V. Kuhnlein, and Olivier Receveur. 2005. "Estimation of Traditional Food Intake in Indigenous Communities in Denendeh and the Yukon." *International Journal of Circumpolar Health* 64 (1): 46–54.

Belinsky, D.K., and Harriet V. Kuhnlein. 2000. "Macronutrient, Mineral, and Fatty Acid Composition of Canada Goose (Branta canadensis): An Important Traditional Food Resource of the Eastern James Bay Cree of Quebec." *Journal of Food Composition and Analysis* 13 (2): 101–15.

Berti, Peter R., Rula Soueida, and Harriet V. Kuhnlein. 2008. "Dietary Assessment of Indigenous Canadian Arctic Women with a Focus on Pregnancy and Lactation." *International Journal of Circumpolar Health* 67 (4): 349–62.

Bishop, Charles A. 1970. The Emergence of Hunting Territories among the Northern Ojibwa. *Ethnology* 9 (1): 1–15.

———. 1984. "The First Century: Adaptive Changes among the Western James Bay Cree between the Early Seventeenth and Early Eighteenth Centuries." In *The Subarctic Fur Trade: Native Social and Economic Adaptations*, edited by Shepard Krech III, 21–54. Vancouver: University of British Columbia Press.

Blanchet, Carole, Eric Dewailly, Pierre Ayotte, Suzanne Bruneau, Olivier Receveur, and B. J. Holub. 2000. "Contribution of Selected Traditional and Market Foods to the Diet of Nunavik Inuit Women." *Canadian Journal of Dietetic Practice and Research* 61 (2): 50–59.

Bruce, Sharon G. 2000. "The Impact of Diabetes Mellitus among the Metis of Western Canada." *Ethnicity and Health* 5 (1): 47–57.

Campbell, Marian L., Ruth M.F. Diamant, Brian D. Macpherson, Judy L. Halladay. 1997. "The Contemporary Food Supply of Three Northern Manitoba Cree Communities." *Canadian Journal of Public Health* 88 (2): 105–08.

Chan, Hing Man, Karen Fediuk, Sue Hamilton, Laura Rostas, Amy Caughey, Harriet V. Kuhnlein, Grace Egeland, and Eric Loring. 2006. "Food Security in Nunavut, Canada: Barriers and Recommendations." *International Journal of Circumpolar Health* 65 (5): 416–31.

Daniel M., K.G. Rowley, C.P. Herbert, K. O'Dea, and L.W. Green. 2001. "Lipids and Psychosocial Status in Aboriginal Persons with and at Risk for Type 2 Diabetes: Implications for Tertiary Prevention." *Patient Education and Counseling* 43 (1): 85–95.

Das, U.N. 2000. "Beneficial Effect(s) of n-3 Fatty Acids in Cardiovascular Diseases: But, Why and How?" *Prostaglandins Leukotrienes and Essential Fatty Acids* 63 (6): 351–62.

Deeb, S.S., L. Fajas, M. Nemoto, J. Pihlajamäki, L. Mykkänen, J. Kuusisto, M. Laakso, W. Fujimoto, and J. Auwerx. 1998. "A Pro12Ala Substitution in PPARgamma2 Associated with Decreased Receptor Activity, Lower Body Mass Index and Improved Insulin Sensitivity." *Nature Genetics* 20 (3): 284–87.

deGonzague, Bernadette, Olivier Receveur, Don Wedll, and Harriet V. Kuhnlein. 1999. "Dietary Intake and Body Mass Index of Adults in 2 Ojibwe Communities. *Journal of the American Dietetic Association* 99 (6): 710–16.

Després, Jean-Pierre, Isabelle Lemieux, Jean Bergeron, Philippe Pibarot, Patrick Mathieu, Eric Larose, Josep Rodés-Cabau, Olivier F. Bertrand, and Paul Poirier. 2008. "Abdominal Obesity and the Metabolic Syndrome: Contribution to Global Cardiometabolic Risk." *Arteriosclerosis, Thrombosis, and Vascular Biology* 28 (6): 1039–49.

Eckel, Robert H., Scott M. Grundy, and Paul Z. Zimmet. 2005. "The Metabolic Syndrome." *Lancet* 365 (9468): 1415–28.

FNIGC (First Nations Information Governance Centre). 2005. *First Nations Regional Longitudinal Health Survey (RHS) 2002/03: The People's report*. Ottawa: First Nations Centre at the National Aboriginal Health Organization (NAHO).

Gillies, Peter J. 2003. "Nutrigenomics: The Rubicon of Molecular Nutrition." *Journal of the American Dietetic Association* 103 (12): S50–55.

Gittelsohn, Joel, Thomas M.S. Wolever, Stewart B. Harris, Robert Harris-Giraldo, Anthony J.G. Hanley, and Bernard Zinman. 1998. "Specific Patterns of Food Consumption and Preparation Are Associated with Diabetes and Obesity in a Native Canadian Community." *Journal of Nutrition* 128 (3): 541–47.

Haman, François, Benedicte Fontaine-Bisson, Malek Batal, Pascal Imbeault, Jules M. Blais, and Michael A. Robidoux. 2010. "Obesity and Type 2 Diabetes in Northern Canada's Remote First Nations Communities: The Dietary Dilemma." *International Journal of Obesity* 34 (S2): S24–S31.

Harris Stewart B., Joel Gittelsohn, Anthony Hanley, Annette Barnie, Thomas M.S. Wolever, Joe Gao, Alexander Logan, and Bernard Zinman. 1997. "The Prevalence of NIDDM and Associated Risk Factors in Native Canadians." *Diabetes Care* 20 (2): 185–87.

Health Canada. 2006. *Canadian Community Health Survey, Cycle 2.2, Nutrition (2004): A Guide to Accessing and Interpreting the Data*. http://www.hc-sc.gc.ca/fn-an/surveill/nutrition/commun/cchs_guide_escc-eng.php.

Hegele, Robert. 1999. "Genetic Prediction of Atherosclerosis: Lessons from Studies in Native Canadian Populations." *Clinica Chimica Acta* 286 (1-2): 47–61.

Hegele, Robert A., Henian Cao, Stewart B. Harris, Bernard Zinman, Anthony J. Hanley, and Carol M. Anderson. 2000. "Peroxisome Proliferator-Activated Receptor-Gamma2 P12A and Type 2 Diabetes in Canadian Oji-Cree." *Journal of Clinical Endocrinology and Metabolism* 85 (5): 2014–19.

Hegele, Robert A., Philip W. Connelly, Anthony J. Hanley, Fang Sun, Stewart B. Harris, and Bernard Zinman. 1997. "Common Genomic Variants Associated with Variation in Plasma Lipoproteins in Young Aboriginal Canadians." *Arteriosclerosis Thrombosis Vascular Biology* 17 (6): 1060–66.

Hegele, Robert A, Stewart B. Harris, Anthony J. Hanley, Stefan Sadikian, Philip W. Connelly, and Bernard Zinman. 1996. "Genetic Variation of Intestinal Fatty Acid-Binding Protein Associated with Variation in Body Mass in Aboriginal Canadians." *Journal of Clinical Endocrinology and Metabolism* 81 (12): 4334–37.

INAC (Indian and Northern Affairs Canada). 2009. Evaluation Reports 2009–2010 to 2013–2014. Ottawa: Government of Canada. http://www.aadnc-aandc.gc.ca/DAM/DAM-INTER-HQ/STAGING/texte-text/ep3_1100100011287_eng.pdf.

Jobling, Mark A. 2012. "The Impact of Recent Events on Human Genetic Diversity." *Philosophical Transactions of the Royal Society B* 367 (1590): 793–99.

Johnson, Suzanne M., David Martin, and Christopher Sarin. 2002. "Diabetes Mellitus in the First Nations Population of British Columbia, Canada. Part 3. Prevalence of Diagnosed Cases." *International Journal of Circumpolar Health* 61 (3): 260–64.

Katzmarzyk, Peter T. 2002. "The Canadian obesity epidemic, 1985-1998." *Canadian Medical Association Journal* 166 (8):1039–40.

———. 2008. "Obesity and Physical Activity among Aboriginal Canadians." *Obesity* 16 (1):184–190.

Kuhnlein, Harriet V. 2004. "Karat, Pulque, and Gac: Three Shining Stars in the Traditional Food Galaxy." *Nutrition Reviews* 62 (11): 439–42.

Kuhnlein, Harriet V., H. M. Chan, D. Leggee, and V. Barthet. 2002. "Macronutrient, Mineral and Fatty Acid Composition of Canadian Arctic Traditional Food." *Journal of Food Composition and Analysis* 15 (5): 545–66.

Kuhnlein, Harriet V. and Olivier Receveur. 2007. "Local Cultural Animal Food Contributes High Levels of Nutrients for Arctic Canadian Indigenous Adults and Children." *Journal of Nutrition* 137 (4): 1110–14.

Kuhnlein, Harriet V., Olivier Receveur, Rula Soueida, and Peter R. Berti. 2008. "Unique Patterns of Dietary Adequacy in Three Cultures of Canadian Arctic Indigenous Peoples." *Public Health Nutrition* 11 (4): 349–60.

Kuhnlein, Harriet V., Rula Soueida, and Olivier Receveur. 1996. "Dietary Nutrient Profiles of Canadian Baffin Island Inuit Differ by Food Source, Season, and Age." *Journal of the American Dietetic Association* 96 (2): 155–62.

Kwon, Y.I., E. Apostolidis, Y.C. Kim, and K. Shetty. 2007. "Health Benefits of Traditional Corn, Beans, and Pumpkin: In Vitro Studies for Hyperglycemia and Hypertension Management." *Journal of Medicinal Food* 10 (2): 266–75.

Lambden, Jill, Olivier Receveur, Joan Marshall, and Harriet V. Kuhnlein. 2006. "Traditional and Market Food Access in Arctic Canada is Affected by Economic Factors." *International Journal of Circumpolar Health* 65 (4): 331–40.

Lear, Scott A., Wei Q. Deng, Guillaume Paré., Dian C. Sulistyoningrum, Ruth J.F. Loos, and Angela Devlin. 2011. "Associations of the FTO rs9939609 Variant with Discrete Body Fat Depots and Dietary Intake in a Multi-Ethnic Cohort." *Genetics Research* 93 (6): 419–26.

Ley, Sylvia H., Robert A. Hegele, Stewart B. Harris, Mary Mamakeesick, Henian Cao, Philip W. Connelly, Joel Gittelsohn, Ravi Retnakaran, Bernard Zinman, and Anthony J. Hanley. 2011. "HnF1A G319S Variant, Active Cigarette Smoking and Incident Type 2 Diabetes in Aboriginal Canadians: A Population-Based Epidemiological Study." *BMC Medical Genetics* 12 (1): 1–1.

Luan, Jian'an, Paul O. Browne, Anne-Helen Harding, David J. Halsall, Stephen O'Rahilly, V.K. Krishna Chatterjee, and Nicholas J. Wareham. 2001. "Evidence for Gene-Nutrient Interaction at the PPAR[gamma] Locus." *Diabetes* 50 (3): 686–89.

Nakano, Tomoko, Karen Fediuk, Norma Kassi, Grace M. Egeland, Harriet V. Kuhnlein. 2005a. "Dietary Nutrients and Anthropometry of Dene/Métis and Yukon Children." *International Journal of Circumpolar Health* 64 (2): 147–56.

———. 2005b. "Food Use of Dene/Métis and Yukon Children." *International Journal of Circumpolar Health* 64 (2): 137–46.

Ordovas, Jose M. and Vincent Mooser. 2004. "Nutrigenomics and Nutrigenetics." *Current Opinion in Lipidology* 15 (2): 101–08.

Pal, Shinjini, François Haman, and Michael A. Robidoux. 2013. "The Costs of Local Food Procurement in Two Northern Indigenous Communities in Canada." *Food and Foodways* 21 (2): 132–52.

Pollex, R.L., Anthony J.G. Hanley, Bernard Zinman, Stewart B. Harris, and Robert A. Hegele. 2006. "Clinical and Genetic Associations with Hypertriglyceridemic Waist in a Canadian Aboriginal Population." *International Journal of Obesity* 30 (3): 484–91.

Ray, Arthur J. 1998. "Periodic Shortages, Native Welfare, and the Hudson's Bay Company, 1670–1930." In *Out of the Background: Readings on Canadian Native History*, edited by Kenneth S. Coates and Robin Fisher, 83–101. Toronto: Irwin Publishing.

Receveur, Olivier, M. Boulay, and Harriet V. Kuhnlein. 1997. "Decreasing Traditional Food Use Affects Diet Quality for Adult Dene/Métis in 16 Communities of the Canadian Northwest Territories." *Journal of Nutrition* 127 (11): 2179–86.

Robidoux, Michael A., François Haman, and Christabelle Sethna. 2009. "The Relationship of the Burbot (Lota lota L.) to the Reintroduction of Off-the-Land Foods in the Sandy Lake First Nation Community." *Biodemography Social Biology* 55 (1):12-29.

Robidoux, Michael A., Malek Batal, Pascal Imbeault, Tim Seabert, Jules M. Blais, Shinjini Pilon, Eva M. Krümmel, and François Haman. 2012. "Traditional Foodways in Two Contemporary Northern First Nations Communities." *Canadian Journal of Native Studies* 32 (1): 59–77.

Robitaille, J., J.P. Després, L. Pérusse, and Marie-Claude Vohl. 2003. The PPAR-gamma P12A Polymorphism Modulates the Relationship between Dietary Fat Intake and Components of the Metabolic Syndrome: Results from the Québec Family Study." *Clinical Genetics* 63 (2): 109–16.

Seabert, Tim, Shinjini Pilon, Eva M. Krümmel, Jules M. Blais, Pascal Imbeault, Michael A. Robidoux, and François Haman. 2013. "Dietary Practices in Isolated First Nations Communities of Northern Canada: Combined Isotopic and Lipid Markers Provide a Good Qualitative Assessment of Store-Bought vs Locally Harvested Foods Consumption. *Nutrition and Diabetes* 3 (10): e92, 1–7.

Simopoulos, Artemis P. 2010. "Nutrigenetics/Nutrigenomics." *Annual Review of Public Health* 31: 53–68.

Solomons, Noel W. 2009. "Developmental Origins of Health and Disease: Concepts, Caveats, and Consequences for Public Health Nutrition." *Nutrition Reviews* 67 (S1): S12–S16.

Szathmáry, Emöke J.E., Cheryl Ritenbaugh, and Carol-Sue M. Goodby. 1987. "Dietary Change and Plasma Glucose Levels in Amerindian Population Undergoing Cultural Transition." *Social Science and Medicine* 24 (10): 791–804.

Tjepkema, Michael. 2006. "Adult Obesity." *Health Reports* 17 (3): 9–25.

Tremblay, Mark S., Peter T. Katzmarzyk, and J.D. Willms. 2002. "Temporal Trends in Overweight and Obesity in Canada, 1981–1996." *International Journal of Obesity* 26 (4): 538–43.

Vanhees Kimberly, Indira G.C. Vonhogen, Frederik J. van Schooten, and Roger W.L. Godschalk. 2014. "You Are What You Eat, and So Are Your Children: The Impact of Micronutrients on the Epigenetic Programming of Offspring." *Cellular and Molecular Life Sciences* 27 (2): 271–85.

Wein, Eleanor E. 1995. "Nutrient Intakes of First Nations People in Four Yukon communities." *Nutrition Research* 15 (8): 1105–19.

Weiss, Mark L., and Justin Tackney. 2012. "An Introduction to Genetics." In *Human Biology: An Evolutionary and Biocultural Perspective*, 2nd edition, edited by Sara Stinson, Barry Bogin, and Dennis O'Rourke, 53–98. Hoboken, NJ: Wiley-Blackwell.

Young, T. Kue. 1994. *The Health of Native Americans: Toward a Biocultural Epidemiology*. New York: Oxford University Press.

Young, T. Kue, Jeff Reading, Brenda Elias, and John D. O'Neil. 2000. "Type 2 Diabetes Mellitus in Canada's First Nations: Status of an Epidemic in Progress." *Canadian Medical Association Journal* 163 (5): 561–66.

Chapter Three

COLLABORATIVE RESPONSES TO REBUILDING LOCAL FOOD AUTONOMY IN THREE INDIGENOUS COMMUNITIES IN NORTHWESTERN ONTARIO

So far, the chapters in this collection have largely focussed on the issues and challenges Indigenous peoples in Northern Ontario encounter as a result of Euro-Canadian intervention and colonization. Through working with Indigenous communities in Sandy Lake, Wapekeka, and Kasabonika Lake, our research group (Indigenous Health Research Group) has tried to understand the impact these changes have had and continue to have on local peoples, in particular on local food systems and the uptake of chronic disease. We have developed comprehensive research programs that explore the extent to which local food sources are harvested and consumed, the differences in health profiles of people who consume local foods versus market foods, and the various health parameters associated with differences in dietary intake (e.g., levels of overweight/obesity, type 2 diabetes, inflammation, fatty acid profiles, and levels of contaminants). The research has led to several peer-reviewed publications and academic or public presentations. They highlight the alarmingly high prevalence of overweight and obesity, the high rate of type 2 diabetes (1 in 3), and the limited access to nutritious foods—whether land-based or store-bought in these communities (Haman et al. 2010; Imbeault et al. 2011; Pal, Haman, and Robidoux 2013). This research draws attention to the health disparities Indigenous peoples in this region encounter and the various factors contributing to these disparities. That said, it was clear early on that our research had very little impact on the communities themselves and that for the most part we did not offer them any new information. Community members were often keenly aware of the increasing prevalence of obesity-related diseases and their tragic health impacts. They were also aware that they did not have regular access to affordable nutritious foods and that it was increasingly difficult to get access to land-based foods for a variety of reasons, such as cost, knowledge, and availability, just to name a few.

As mentioned in the introduction, our research program was fortuitously adapted in 2009 as a result of a funding opportunity made available by the Canadian Partnership Against Cancer (CPAC). Through various research networks, our group was invited to participate in a unique project—one that was purposefully designed to bring about collaborations between researchers, practitioners, policy makers, and communities—to work toward preventing chronic disease. The initiative created by CPAC was to fund a series of Coalitions Linking Action and Science for Prevention (CLASP) projects over a three-year period. Working with a coalition led by the Chronic Disease Prevention Alliance of Canada, our research group assisted in developing one of the seven CLASP projects. Our project was titled Collaborative Action on Childhood Obesity (CACO). Our role was to bring Indigenous partners, with whom we were already working, into the project and to provide them with resources for local land-based programming. In turn, our Indigenous partners were to use these resources to build local food capacity and increase food availability and quality—with the overall objective of preventing obesity/chronic disease. I will present the results of this initiative. Through this project, the participating Indigenous communities were able to increase their community land-based programming and food procurement, and we learned the implications of community-based research and gained insights into working with Indigenous communities. Together, we saw the potential of local food procurement in preventing obesity-related chronic disease in remote northern Indigenous communities.

Community Engagement

At the outset of this project, our group was already in partnership with two remote Indigenous communities in Northwestern Ontario: Wapekeka First Nation and Kasabonika Lake First Nation. We were just concluding a contaminant study, funded by Health Canada's First Nations Environmental Contaminants Program, and we informed these communities about the unique CLASP initiative. We saw that this funding opportunity could move beyond research and support land-based programs that were already informally running in these communities, on an ad hoc basis. Both communities expressed interest in applying for the funds, as did a smaller community, Wawakapewin, which was part of the same tribal council as Kasabonika Lake and Wapekeka. We had presented our findings from previous projects to the entire Shibogama Tribal Council the year before, and members from the Wawakapewin First Nation expressed interest in the work and in potential collaborations. As covered in great detail in Chapter 4, their interest, however, was not exactly the same as the other communities'. The Wawakapewin community felt that to increase land-based food harvesting it was necessary to build a land-based education program, which provided youth with the necessary skills to get on the land and learn to hunt and to prepare foods as their ancestors had. While not dramatically different, their concerns did move outside of our immediate objective of increasing food access for remote Indigenous communities to help in the prevention of obesity and obesity-related diseases.

Wawakapewin's interest in working with us posed a significant challenge in that we needed to accommodate what the community was requesting while maintaining a focus that satisfied the grant requirements. Wawakapewin's participation also marked an important change in how we began to think about, and approach, community-based research. Grounded in more classical research perspectives, our group typically approached communities with questions we thought communities might be interested in, as opposed to communities coming to us with questions and issues they wanted resolved. In this case, it was made clear at the outset of the collaboration that participation was contingent on each community having ownership of its project, on each community's unique interests being met, and on the research group conducting the projects according to community protocols. Land-based programming and food procurement was at the core of all the projects, but each community envisioned distinctive strategies in achieving programming goals. After in-person meetings with community leaders and tribal council officials, we were able to frame the project around building capacity through land-based food procurement—whether it involved infrastructure development, training and education, or providing funds for the actual food harvesting and preparation. In turn, each community was tasked with developing its own project plan, based on any of these three components (independent of one another or in combination), and with providing us with a list of project activities as well as a budget required to complete them. In total we secured approximately $415,000 for the communities to split three ways over the two-and-a-half-year duration of the project.

Project Rationale

Prior to discussing each community's land-based program, it is imperative to provide context for each community and explain why efforts and resources were directed toward the development of certain types of programming. The three communities are located in the northwestern interior of Ontario, roughly 600 kilometres north of Thunder Bay. They are fly-in communities with no road access, except during the coldest months of winter when a winter road is constructed. Kasabonika and Wapekeka have small airports, which allow for regularly scheduled passenger and freight flights, whereas Wawakapewin does not have an airport and planes must land on water or the ice when conditions permit. As a result, the costs to ship goods from the South to these remote communities are exceptional, making it extremely expensive to buy even the most basic household items, including food. The Northern Food Basket research (Indian and Northern Affairs Canada 2006), comparing grocery prices from urban Canadian centres to those in remote Indigenous communities, indicates that food costs were in some cases over 50 percent higher in the North. For example, in 2006 a week's worth of food basket perishables (e.g., milk, eggs, vegetables) in Thunder Bay cost $58, whereas in Fort Severn, a community northeast of Wapekeka, the same basket cost $119. The results were equally alarming when considering nonperishable food items. The nonperishable food basket (e.g., rice, dry pasta) estimates in Thunder Bay came in at $87, compared to Fort Severn at $157 (ibid.).

One of the critiques of food basket research is its southern urban bias that fails to consider market alternatives (e.g., wild game and wild edible plants), which make up an important part of the diet of people living in northern Indigenous communities. Taking this into consideration, our group (Pal, Haman, and Robidoux 2013) documented costs associated with hunting and fishing in Kasabonika Lake and Wapekeka First Nations and compared these costs to market food pricing. While there was a significant range in costs associated with hunting and fishing depending on where these activities took place, the research indicated that: "The average cost of meat from the land was noted as $14.32/kg, which is higher than the cost of store meats (which ranges from $6 to $11). Nevertheless some of these foods, depending on the distance travelled to harvest them, are comparable in cost to store foods. Depending on the type of meat procured (mostly moose, as mentioned earlier) the cost can range instead from $1 to $9/kg" (ibid., 144).

The main conclusion from our research was that in both of these communities, whether market or land-based, food costs are exorbitant, and with the high rates of unemployment and poverty in Kasabonika Lake and Wapekeka, it is virtually impossible to consume a healthy diet.

The health costs of poor nutrition and limited food access have been well documented in Indigenous communities across Canada (Willows 2005; Burnett, Skinner, and LeBlanc 2015). These studies repeatedly indicate a disproportionately higher burden of chronic disease in Indigenous compared to non-Indigenous Canadian communities (Anand et al. 2001; Haman et al. 2010; Young et al. 2000). Research specific to Kasabonika Lake and Wapekeka First Nations (Imbeault et al. 2011) was conducted by our group from 2009 to 2010 and documented the prevalence of overweight/ obesity and the incidence of type 2 diabetes among adult men and women. The results from this study revealed numbers that exceed not only Canadian national averages but Canadian Indigenous national averages as well. According to the First Nations Regional Health Survey 2008/10, the prevalence of overweight and obesity of First Nations peoples living on reserve in 2002–03 was approximately 73 percent. In comparison, non-Indigenous peoples in Canada were reported to have a prevalence of overweight and obesity of approximately 50 percent (FNIGC 2012). For those adults sampled in the Kasabonika Lake and Wapekeka First Nations the prevalence of overweight and obesity was 91.6 percent. Within the same population sample, it was reported that 36.1 percent were considered type 2 diabetic, which grossly exceeds the 8.3 percent average for non-Indigenous Canadians within the same age range (Imbeault et al. 2011). These numbers are of grave concern and, with high food costs and limited availability of healthy food options, the prognosis for improvement is not good. Moreover, based on the remote locations of the communities and limited impact current government subsidies are having on importing food (see Pal, Haman, and Robidoux 2013), a more local response to address these issues is necessary. It is in this context that the Collaborative Action on Childhood Obesity (CACO) project emerged. With substantive funding, these three communities in Northern Ontario were able to work toward building greater food capacity and to procure local food sources to supplement what was available in stores. In the following section, I provide details about each community's project and what its members accomplished during the funding period.

Kasabonika Lake First Nation

Kasabonika Lake First Nation is an Oji-Cree community located on the Asheweig River, approximately thirty kilometres south of Wapekeka. It is the largest of the three communities with a population of approximately 914 band members with the majority of them (866) living on reserve. The community has one major store, the Northern Store, and some smaller confectionary stores that have limited produce and groceries but a wide variety of junk foods (pop, chips, and candy). There is an elementary and secondary school, an arena, and a fully equipped nursing station. As in the other two communities, the main languages spoken are Oji-Cree and English.

The programming that was initiated in Kasabonika Lake focussed on training youth land-based harvesting and food preparation skills, on procuring and preparing wild food, and on developing a community garden. Each community had complete control over how the funds were spent, as long as the money was utilized in setting up or running of their program. In Kasabonika, a large percentage of the funding was spent on transportation costs of getting on the land to hunt and freight costs to bring back food to the community. Funds were also spent on hunting equipment and outdoor clothing, which is extremely expensive and is a real deterrent for people wishing to get on the land, especially in the colder winter months. On longer trips only hunters with sufficient skills would participate, in part due to costs of travel but also for safety reasons. For shorter day trips, youth would accompany hunters and Elders to learn first-hand how to navigate the land, how to handle the equipment (transportation and hunting tools), how to hunt or fish, and how to prepare the animals once harvested. When food was brought back to the community, food was either prepared and stored for public feasts and community gatherings, or delivered directly to households with residents who were unable to partake in community gatherings for health-related reasons. If large yields were gathered, women would organize at a local teepee and they would collectively prepare the food. On one occasion I attended, for example, over 300 geese were prepared. *Kookums* (grandmothers in Oji-Cree) from various families came together at one Elder's backyard teepee and began plucking geese, treating the birds, and singeing the carcasses over a fire in the teepee and outside in the yard. Multiple generations gathered and interacted with the women as the work was being carried out. A call was put out over the radio and community members were able to come and pick up one goose per family. Birds that were not picked up were placed in community freezers (which were purchased with project funds) and kept for community feasts, held routinely throughout the year.

It was determined at the outset of the project that an intergenerational approach would be utilized to teach land-based skills during all project activities. Through this intergenerational approach, Elders, hunters, and those experienced in preparing food taught youth a wide range of skills that are critical for the acquisition of wild game and its preparation, but also for surviving on the land. The working group responsible for the Kasabonika Lake project identified activities for the spring harvest, the teachings associated with each activity, and what was achieved as a result of the activity (see Table 3.1). The costs for these activities totalled $32,711. As evident from the contents of the table, food harvesting in the spring primarily involved goose hunting and fishing. However, during any hunting event, other forms of wild game were harvested when opportunities presented themselves (as seen with the beaver, moose, and caribou). There were two types of hunting trips: one type that involved air travel to a major goose-hunting area near Fort Severn, located on the southwestern shore of Hudson Bay; and the other that involved local trips made by boat, all-terrain vehicles

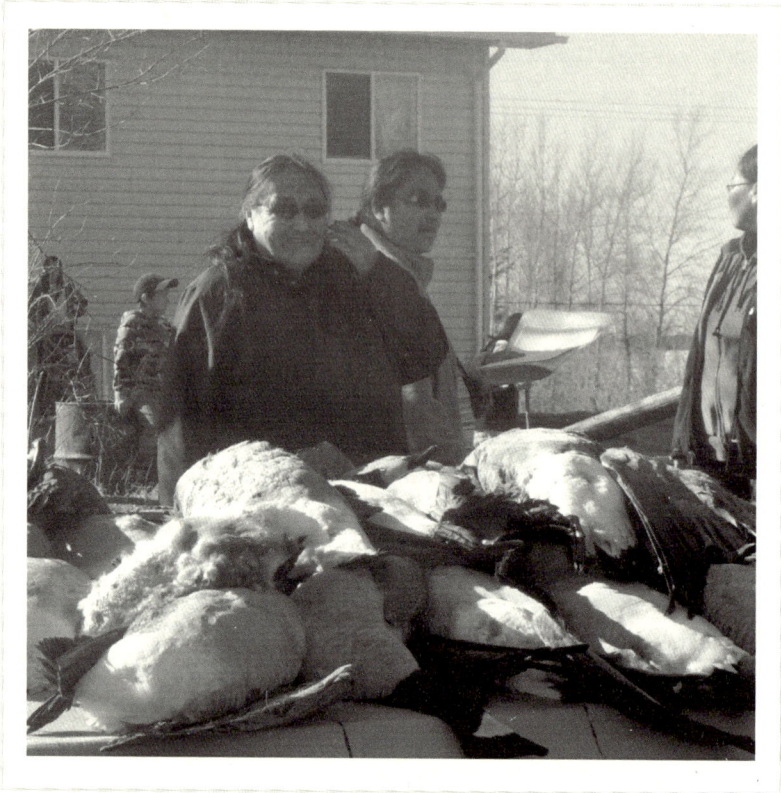

Figure 3.1. Geese distribution after spring hunt in the Kasabonika Lake First Nation. Photograph by Michael A. Robidoux.

(quads), or snowmobiles, depending on the season. These organized hunts brought in considerable yields to supplement regular and local hunting and fishing activities, and provided fresh meat for community members who were unable to get on the land.

The information provided in the table also highlights the costs, efforts, and knowledge involved in procuring wild game. The project funds covered important material costs that allowed more trips and more people to get on the land, but the yearly operational costs, including fuel and flights, remained high. The level of effort involved in tracking, successfully hunting or fishing, and preparing wild game is considerable, and not everyone is able to invest time or money to do it on a regular basis. Recognizing

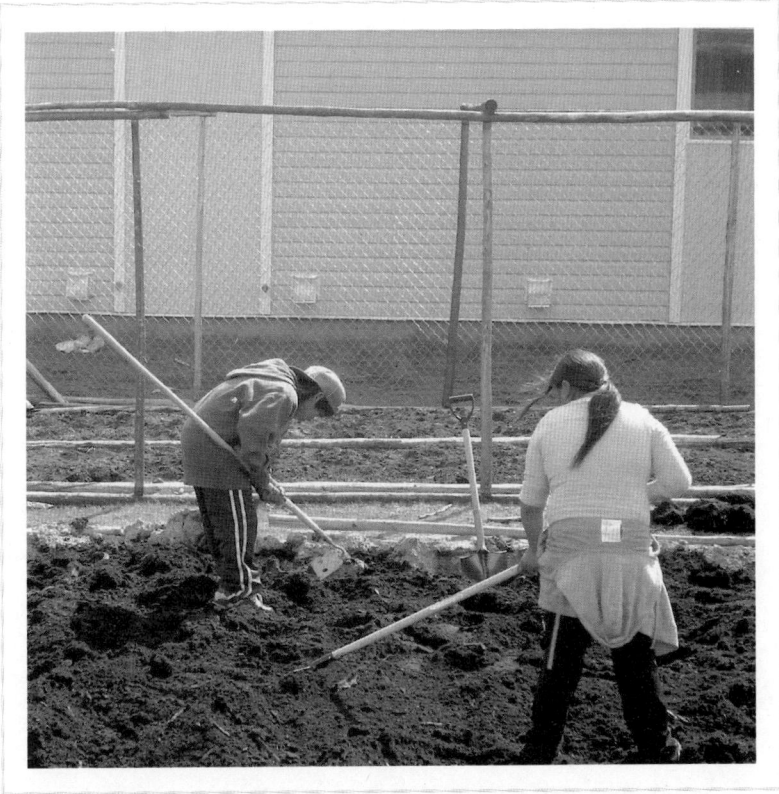

Figure 3.2. Youth helping prepare soil for early stages of community garden development in Kasabonika Lake First Nation. Photograph by Michelle Kehoe.

these challenges, the community-working group requested to add another component to their project, which was the development of a community garden. The proposed garden was not intended to minimize or reduce more traditional harvesting activities, but to supplement local food supplies. By locally producing fruits and vegetables, the community could increase access to nutritional content that wild game[1] does not provide, and increase it at a cost significantly lower than hunting and fishing.

Oji-Cree communities in this region have always cultivated wild edible plants, but only after permanent settlements were established post-1930 did formal Western gardening techniques get introduced, largely through Christian missionaries. Elders in Kasabonika remember potato gardens in

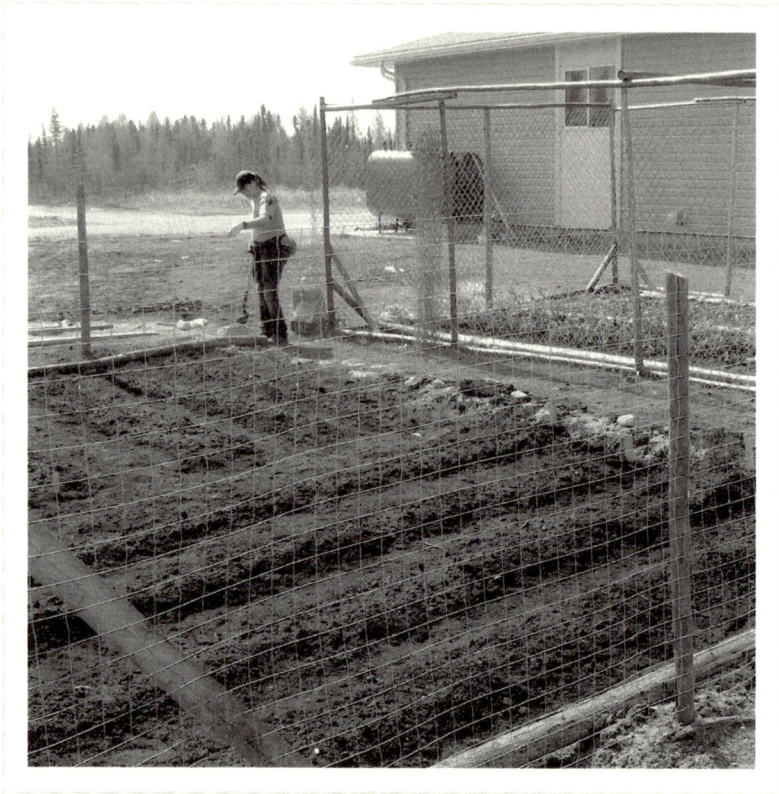

Figure 3.3. First day of planting at Kasabonika Lake First Nation community garden.
Photograph by Mélanie St-Jean.

the old settlement (the community was relocated in the 1960s), but there
has been little to no gardening since then. Therefore the working group
knew very little about gardens, about how to set one up or about what could
grow in their community. Despite these challenges, they decided to construct a garden by utilizing knowledge acquired over the internet and by
using the minimal resources provided by our CACO project. They decided
to build the garden next to the Elders' Complex with the assistance of the
Community Prevention Coordinator and University of Ottawa students,
who were documenting project activities as part of their graduate degrees.
With less than $3,000 of supplies the project team created two fenced-in

ACTIVITY	SUPPLIES NEEDED	TEACHINGS	YIELDS & OUTCOMES
Canadian Geese and Snow Geese Harvest in Fort Severn (10-Day Trip)	14 cases of ammunition (shotgun shells) Chartered flights to Fort Severn Freight delivery to and from camp Cabins/Lodgings		700+ geese
Local Hunting Trips	Quads (4) Boats and motors (4) Gill nets (4) Gas Oil Chain oil Tarps Rope Tea bags Coffee Milk Flour Oats Plastic cutlery, Styrofoam cups and plates	Survival skills Promoting healthy lifestyle living to community members Portaging rapids How to set up fish nets, traps Gun safety Learning and listening to the elderly people Teaching skills and knowledge from the Elders What clothes to wear when going hunting and fishing (in snow or rain)	300+ geese 5 beaver 50+ ducks 2 moose 2 caribou 250+ families were fed and taught during these 2 months
Food Preparation	Cut wood 2 teepees Gloves Garbage bags Ziploc bags	Site preparation for spring food harvest Maintaining and cleaning the site where the traditional preparation is done How to singe the geese Hands-on teaching from the elderly people Filleting the fish How to cook the traditional food How to smoke traditional foods How to clean traditional foods How to preserve foods traditionally and through freezer and/or refrigeration	100+ youth were involved by listening and looking at the teachings of the elderly women and men

Table 3.1. Land-Based Project Activities at Kasabonika Lake First Nation.
Information in this table is a synthesis of the Kasabonika Lake First Nation community coordinator report highlighting program activities, costs, and outcomes over a six-month period.

garden spaces approximately 3 x 5 m and 4 x 7 m. They planted tomatoes, potatoes, green onions, green beans, carrots, and strawberries (Kasabonika Fiscal Period 5 Report, April 2012). According to one community member who was involved with constructing and maintaining the garden, "We had lots of tomatoes, lots of potatoes, lots of green onions and lots of strawberries. We didn't think anything would come out of it, but it did. So now there is an interest; [community members] are talking about growing their own garden" (April 2012).

Wapekeka First Nation

Wapekeka (Angling Lake) First Nation is located seventy-one kilometres northwest of Kasabonika Lake. The population is composed of approximately 363 band members with the majority (328) living on reserve. The reserve size is 5,566 hectares. Like Kasabonika Lake, Wapekeka is accessible year-round by air and during the winter months by a road constructed over snow and ice. The community has modern housing, running water, and either electric heating, wood stove heating, or a combination of the two. In addition to standard appliances—fridge, stove, washing machine, and dryer—many homes have satellite television and computers with internet connections. Unlike in Kasabonika, in Wapekeka the school only goes up to grade eight, which means that children must leave the community to attend high school—typically in Sioux Lookout or Thunder Bay. Wapekeka has a nursing clinic rather than a nursing station, and a community-owned store rather than a Northern Store. It also has smaller convenience stores, with limited groceries but a constant supply of chips, pop, candy, and other types of junk food.

The project plan developed by Wapekeka community leaders initially focussed on training youth on how to get on the land and how to hunt, fish, and prepare the animals once they were harvested. The leaders identified this as a priority because fewer youth are on the land with parents or grandparents and because many adults do not have the knowledge and financial means to get on the land themselves. As a result, the youth are not acquiring the necessary skills to navigate the land or the extensive waterway systems that permit travel in a region without roads. Some youth are also not learning how to hunt, fish, or prepare the wild meat. The money provided through the grant was used to get youth to join hunters on the land, on local excursions and during overnight camps. This way they learned first-hand how to get on the land, how to use the equipment, how to set up camp, how to hunt and fish, how to give thanks for what the land provides, and how to prepare the animals. In the second year the project developed another component, which was funded through another opportunity secured by the Chronic Disease Prevention Alliance of Canada and the University of Ottawa's Indigenous Health Research Group from the Public Health Agency of Canada. The grant application was written in response to project team members from Wapekeka wishing to cultivate a community garden—to complement the traditional food procurement initiatives established under the CLASP project. Interest in the garden was tremendous and in one short summer, garden production exceeded everyone's expectations. This component has become an integral part of community efforts to gain greater autonomy over food availability and food quality.

Akin to what was proposed in Kasabonika, the Wapekeka project focussed on activities that intended to increase food yields for the community and also provided opportunities for youth to learn from hunters how to get on the land and how to engage in land-based procurement. The following table, provided by the community coordinator in Wapekeka, outlines the types of activities conducted during the spring and summer months in the first year of the project, the knowledge shared through each activity, as well as the estimated costs.

Wapekeka is fortunate to have a group of people interested in maintaining traditional cultural practices, whether it be in the arts and crafts, making clothing like moccasins, hats, and mittens, or in getting on the land, harvesting food and preparing it in traditional ways. One family in particular has taken a leadership role in this regard, by providing a physical space where teaching can occur and by organizing cultural programming whenever possible. Such programming requires considerable knowledge and resources, as is evident in the tables above. The Wapekeka community is well equipped with knowledge bearers, but constantly struggles to get funding to support cultural programs. The CACO project allowed the community to build strategic infrastructure and make material purchases to get youth on the land and participating in harvesting activities, but it also

ACTIVITY	SUPPLIES NEEDED	TEACHINGS	COSTS
Thursday, 13 May to Tuesday, 18 May, 2010 Otter Lake—duck, geese, and beaver hunting (34 miles from Wapekeka) 9 hunters 3 boats in Otter Lake	12 cases of shells (ammunition) Groceries Fuel (405 litres) Outboard oil Gear oil for outboard motors Tarp Candles Coleman stove fuel Chainsaw oil Garbage bags	Clean and prepare the ducks, geese, and beaver Prepare the beaver for smoking Keeping ducks/geese/beaver cold by digging a hole in the ground (permafrost) and using moss and pine branches to cover the area Gun cleaning and gun safety Make a duck blind Repair and clean an outboard motor, and change the gear oil Maintain and clean up the campsite Set up the fish net, how to take fish, and how to prepare/cook the fish	$ 10,863.70
Wednesday, 9 June to Sunday, 13 June, 2010 Otter Lake and Otter River—Sturgeon net fishing and moose hunting 7 hunters Travel by float plane to Otter Lake and by 3 boats to Otter River	Sinkers and floaters for all 7 nets (20 each) Gas (354 litres) Oil (8) Stove fuel (2) Groceries Blue twine (3) Black twine (3)	Setting up fish nets in the river Mend the nets Installing floaters and sinkers on the nets Hanging and storing fish nets Preserving the sturgeon in the water Butchering the sturgeon Boat safety, navigating the river Motor/boat maintenance Making a tent frame, preparing a campsite Butcher and debone a moose for travel, dispose of the guts, respect the animal, smoke the meat Gun safety	$ 5,422.65
19–20 June, 2010 Youth camping trip to Big Trout Lake 4 boats 4 youth and 4 chaperones	Gas (198 litres) Oil (5) Groceries	Fish using a fishing rod, i.e., trolling for walleye and trout Cast the rod and remove the hook from fish Portage through the rapids Boat safety Fillet the fish Set up a tent Prepare and maintain campsites What types of clothes to wear when fishing/hunting under various conditions Make a fire and put it out thoroughly Operate the outboard motor	$ 882.73
August 2010 Otter River Hunting and taking Gas (198 litres) in preparation for the fall moose hunt 3 boats 6 hunters	Gas (462 litres) Oil (11) Groceries Naphtha/fuel Camp stoves Rifle, ammunition Sandbags	Using an outboard motor, boat safety, and motor maintenance Travelling through the waterway, navigating big rocks, reefs, and rapids Moose hunting and calling Butcher and debone a moose for travel, dispose of the guts, respect the animal, smoke the meat Snare a moose	$5,500.00

Table 3.2. Land-Based Project Activities at Wapekeka First Nation.
Information in this table is a synthesis of the Wapekeka First Nation community coordinator report highlighting program activities, costs, and outcomes over a six-month period.

enabled the hunters to provide for their community by distributing their yields through expanded food-sharing networks.

Prior to the CACO project, hunters would bring back wild game and distribute it amongst family and friends. The resources from the grant, however, enabled the community to implement a more formalized food-sharing system that went beyond these informal networks. This was the community's key objective. There were three modes of food distribution implemented as a result of the project, some expanding on existing processes, others newly introduced. One method, expanded from existing distribution methods, was to simply announce over the community radio that hunters were coming in with harvested meat. This way people were able to come to a central place in the community and pick up a portion. The site was a log house a community member built to serve as a cultural resource centre. The hunters would bring the meat there and it would be collectively prepared. As will be discussed at length in Chapter 5, it was most often the female Elders that played a lead role in this process. After the preparation, the meat would be laid out across the floor and on tables, and people would show up, usually visit, and then return home with some of the meat. On some occasions a feast would be arranged from what was harvested and a call would go out on the radio, inviting anyone to come and have a prepared meal. Some people would sit and eat the meal together in the log house, while others would come, pick up their meal, and return home or deliver it to a family member who was not able to attend. These were highly social activities that provided rich intergenerational interaction and positive engagement amongst community members. The food sharing was also an opportunity to give thanks to the hunters who provided the meat and the women who predominantly prepared it.

There are, however, limitations to this form of distribution in that it draws on existing food-sharing networks rather than creating new ones. This is not to suggest that people were excluded from the invitation, but that there is a certain level of comfort required to come to this central place and to take the food that is offered. The Wapekeka community is small and relatively tight-knit, and there are traditional clan lines that do influence the levels of social interaction between families, including how food would have traditionally been shared. For this reason, the same people

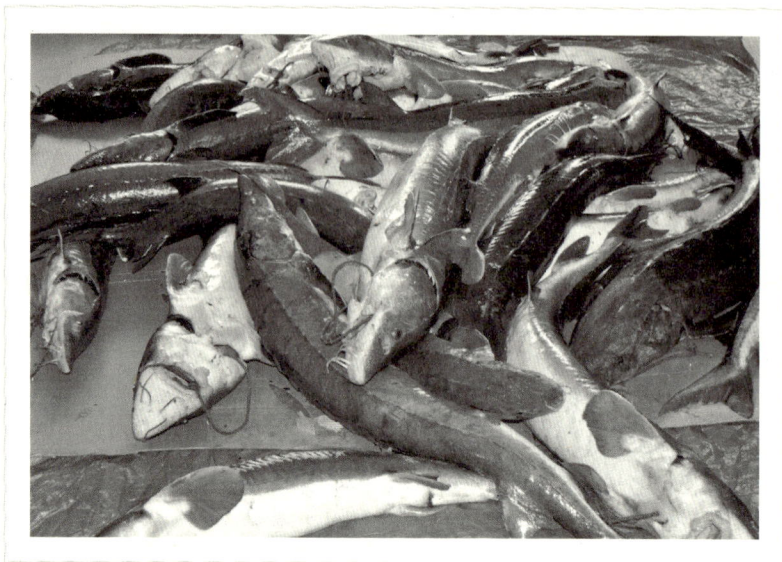

Figure 3.4. Wapekeka First Nation log house with sturgeon placed on the floor to be cleaned and packaged for storage/distribution. Photograph by Shinjini Pilon.

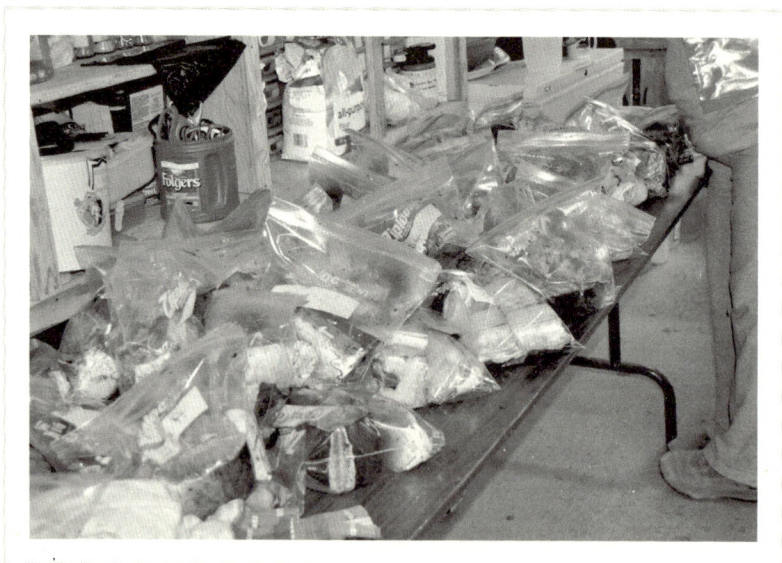

Figure 3.5. Food being packaged and made ready for community distribution in Wapekeka First Nation. Photograph by Shinjini Pilon.

often attended these types of food-sharing occasions. Out of community concern, new alternative methods to distribute food to others, who were not taking advantage of the open call system, were devised. The first and easiest way was to hold public feasts in other settings than the log house so people without any direct associations to it would feel comfortable attending. New feast sites were constructed on the community's waterfront, which provided inviting settings for people to gather and share meals. Another important dimension to public feasts was to utilize locally procured foods whenever possible. The use of wild game has always been a part of feasts, but with the development of the community garden, local fruits and vegetables were being served as well. This added a whole new source of pride to the meals and created further autonomy over the local food system.

The final food distribution method developed through the project was likely the least successful, but interestingly reveals the level of commitment to the project and how much the project organizers wanted it to work. Even with the public feasts taking place in more neutral spaces in the community, it was evident that not all community members were taking advantage of the foods being made available. According to the main project lead, Clara Winnepetonga, those not participating were some of the more disadvantaged people in the community. They had the fewest resources to buy food or to go on the land and procure food for themselves. In order to maximize food distribution efforts, individuals went door to door with small parcels of food that were prepared and packaged when hunters returned with their catch. Whether it was fish or wild game, the meat was prepared in the log house, put in freezer bags, and then distributed door to door throughout the community.

This mode of food distribution, however, had limited success for two important reasons. First, it required a massive amount of food to be equally distributed across approximately fifty homes. Second, there were concerns that, in some isolated cases, the food was not being consumed by members of the household, but sold for temporary and minimal economic gain. There were allegations that some community members were selling the food to support an oxycodone addiction, which had become a serious problem in the community at the time of this project. When the hunters and community project leaders learned that the food was being sold, they were extremely disheartened and immediately discontinued this service.

Instead, the community responded with an initiative that turned out to be one of the remarkable success stories of the CACO project.

Wapékeka, like many other communities in this region of Northwestern Ontario, was struggling with the devastating effects of oxycodone addiction. The Nishnawbe Aski Nation (NAN) estimated that upwards of 10,000 people in the region were suffering from addictions and that communities were undergoing a serious crisis (Canadian Press 2012). Health Canada responded by banning oxycodone production and sale in Canada, which did make it more difficult to obtain, but as a result created a host of other problems. There was the serious physical pain of sudden opiate withdrawal and many people in the community were left to suffer without proper medical resources. Moreover, the limited supply raised oxycodone's street value, which triggered desperate behaviour from those addicted to the drug. Communal and individual safety was at risk—homes were being broken into, family members were victimized, and some individuals resorted to prostitution to get enough money to purchase whatever little of the drug was available. The backlash was as traumatic as the addiction itself. NAN issued a news release at the time Health Canada banned the drug, and its deputy grand chief Mike Metatawabin stated: "We have a public health catastrophe on our hands and no one is stepping up to take responsibility to help our people. . . . Our communities have minimal access to medical service to help cope with severe withdrawal symptoms. Our people have a right to timely and effective health care" (NAN 2012, para. 4). In the press release, NAN officials were looking for "culturally relevant and community based treatment" along with land-based programming "to work on root causes of addiction" (ibid., para. 8). Health Canada has since provided initial funding for a suboxone opiate replacement therapy, and its early results are showing to be extremely effective (CBC News 2014). Community leaders in Wapekeka, however, did not wait to see if and when the federal government would respond. They began taking people suffering from addictions onto the land to participate in their own land-based food program as a form of detoxification and therapy.

The land-based therapy program was organized with the community's chief and council, health director, and the hunters who were leading the land-based food programs. Two individuals who had been seeking help for

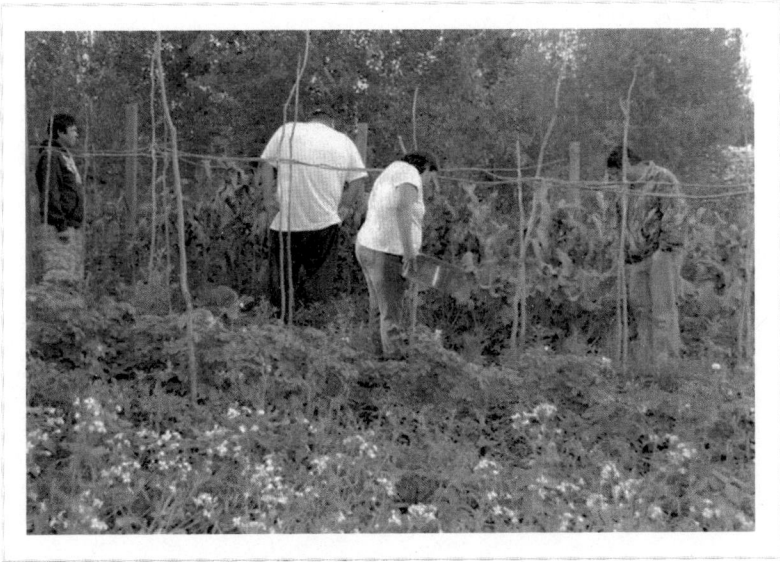

Figure 3.6. Clara Winnepetonga and her family working in the community garden in Wapekeka First Nation. Photograph by Shinjini Pilon.

their addiction were asked to participate in a three-week hunting and fishing expedition. According to project team members, the participants were initially quite sick, as they were going through withdrawal symptoms, and slept most of the first two days. By the third day they started participating in light chores, helping with the fire and with some of the cooking, and slowly began gaining back their strength. By the end of the trip they were fully involved in all activities and were positively connecting with everyone at the camp, with the land, and with their culture. The participants were deeply moved by the experience and did not want to leave for two reasons: one, they felt good being on the land; and two, they were nervous to return to the community setting where their addiction problems first started. Without any aftercare programming, there was little in place to prevent the two participants from returning to the same environment and from facing the same pressures that led to the addictions. The community project members did their best to be there for the people who went through the land-based healing program, but the need for formalized aftercare remained a pressing concern. Two years after Wapekeka initiated their land-based healing

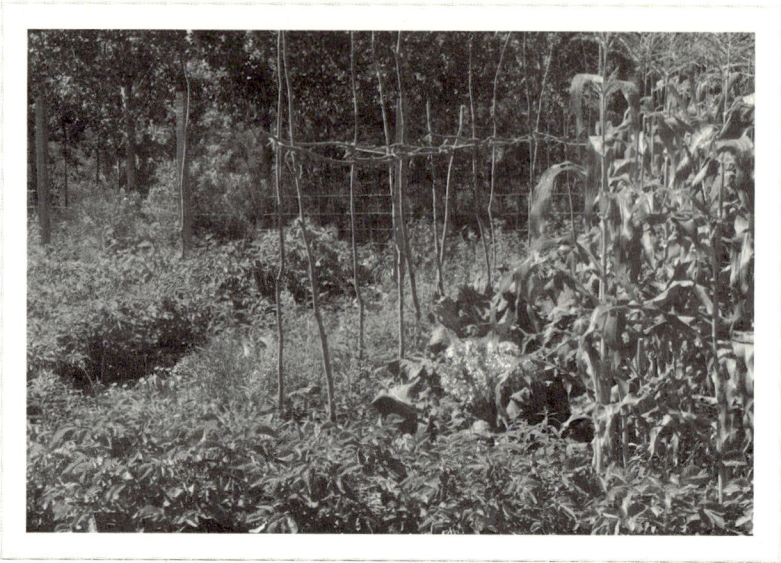

Figure 3.7. Wapekeka community garden at the end of the first summer.
Photograph by Shinjini Pilon.

program, the community was successful in getting a suboxone program through funding from Health Canada. With this program, health professionals took on the suboxone treatment and the land-based healing was more fittingly utilized as the aftercare component, which continues to this day in the community.

The second major component of the Wapekeka project was the development of the community garden. In part supported by additional funds from the Public Health Agency of Canada and the Get Growing Fund from the Nishnawbe Aski Nation, the community garden initiative in Wapekeka has become an inspirational story in the region. The interest largely stemmed from Clara Winnepetonga who, with the assistance of extended family members, was able to construct a large community garden (approximately 7 x 15 m) on a plot of land on the outskirts of the community. Seeds and seedlings were purchased based on taste or preference and according to what was expected to grow in this northern region of Ontario. With assistance from our project team members, the ground was prepared and seeds and seedlings were planted. During this process, some of our team was able to provide knowledge about soil preparation, advice how to grow the various fruits and vegetables that were planted, and information on what was required to maintain the garden throughout the summer. In the first summer the garden was a huge success, producing corn, squash, peas, potatoes, onions, strawberries, and various types of lettuce.

Clara's family was predominantly responsible for the initial startup of the garden, but others became more involved once it started to develop. Children from the community would come and help weed and water the garden. In the first year, water was manually hauled from the lake, which is about fifty metres away from the garden. In year two, the garden was doubled in size and a pump was installed to provide a regular and less labour-intensive water supply. There were challenges throughout, such as snow and sub-zero temperatures partway through the growing season and a cutworm problem in year two, which decimated most of the harvest. The success of the garden, however, proved to be greater than the food that was produced. The garden demonstrated the potential for locally producing fruits and vegetables, which are rarely available in stores and are often of poor quality. It has also become an important success story profiled in the local media, prompting other communities to develop their own community gardens (Garrick 2011). Clara has since been involved in the NAN Food Sovereignty Advisory Group and is an important contributor to the NAN Annual Food Symposium. Finally, the garden has been important in exposing community members to the fresh taste of fruits and vegetables, and in a much broader variety. The garden does not simply make these food sources available in the community for the first time, it increases their palatability, making them more desirable and more likely to be consumed. In combination with the increased harvesting and distribution of wild foods (fish, birds, and land mammals), the project team implemented a local food strategy that had an immediate impact on improving community access to culturally meaningful and healthy foods.

Wawakapewin First Nation

Wawakapewin is the smallest of the three communities and is unique in comparison to the others in many ways. First, unlike Kasabonika and Wapekeka, Wawakapewin is a recently formed community, only receiving official reserve status in 1998. Families that once lived in this territory, prior to the permanent settlement process that was developed through Treaty 9 (and treaty adhesions in the 1930s), sought to reclaim their traditional lands and were successfully recognized as a band in the 1980s. In 1985 the community was granted reserve status. There are only sixty-seven registered band members and only a fraction of those live in the community year-round. There is no airport, which means travel in and out of the community is expensive and limited. Float planes can land on water or ice to deliver supplies and to transport people, but during periods of freeze-up and breakup (between four and six weeks in total) planes are not able to land. Residents are therefore required to be as self-sufficient as possible, ordering food in bulk and procuring as much food from the land as possible. There is no medical office or nursing station, and people must fly out of the community to receive medical attention. This adds to the community's vulnerability during breakup or freeze-up as residents are unable to leave during these periods. These challenges, however, have required Wawakapewin people to develop their own community food strategy in their CACO project plan. In it they identified local food procurement (which involved hunting, fishing, and garden development), regularized food distribution, and land-based teaching as three priority areas.

The land-based food procurement initiatives that the community-project team organized in Wawakapewin were to support existing hunting and fishing activities, but special emphasis was placed on seasonal gatherings that are important occasions for food harvesting and teaching. According to Wawakapewin Elder Simon Frogg, there are six seasons in Oji-Cree culture and the community organizes community gatherings associated with each. The season right after the ice breakup is referred to as Minookum and it is a critical harvesting period, especially for fish. While Minookum is described at length in Chapter 4, it is important to briefly profile it here. The CACO project funds were utilized for building infrastructure at the traditional site, where the gatherings were held, and for buying equipment and tools to optimize land-based activities. The funds also enabled greater participation from those who have ancestral ties to the people from Wawakapewin. People from neighbouring communities like Kasabonika Lake, Wunnumin, and Kingfisher Lake would attend and share in the teachings that Wawakapewin Elders provide. The people in

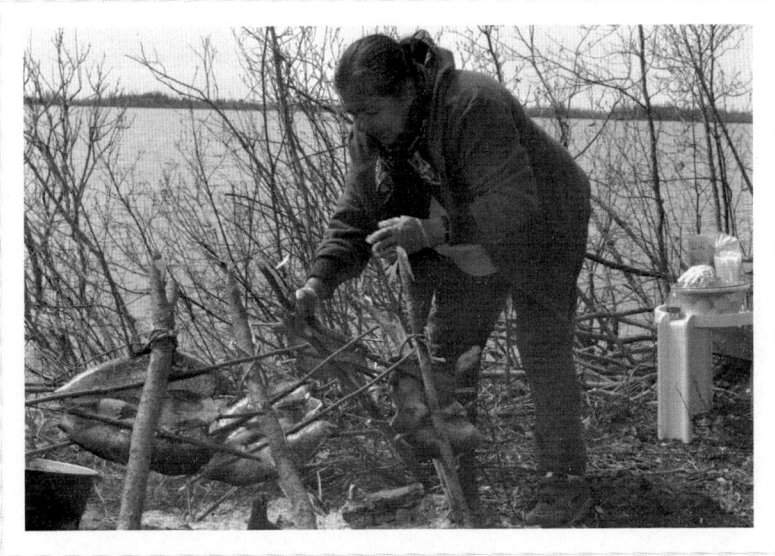

Figure 3.8. Elder at Minookum preparing and drying fish over fire.
Photograph by Michelle Kehoe.

this community are renowned for their knowledge of the land and of traditional cultural practices, in particular those regarding plants and healing.
In addition to collectively harvesting food, Minookum is an intergenerational knowledge-sharing event. At such time, Elders and other tradition
bearers teach people about how wild game, birds, and fish were traditionally harvested, the various methods of food preparation, plants and their
nutritional and medicinal purposes, the legends of their people and the
land, and the people's history in this territory. The teachings are designed,
in part, to stress the value of ancestral ways as a means of becoming more
self-reliant and sustainable, rather than relying exclusively on resources
from the South. Also, these teachings valorize the cultural practices that
have been eroded by Euro-Canadian contact in its multiplicity of mani-
festations. For the Wawakapewin community project leaders, steps toward
improving community health begin with cultural awakenings and learning
about what made their people strong and healthy in the past. Community
gatherings were a starting point to put other physical practices into action.

First a centre was developed to process and store food for collective distribution. Money from the project was used to refurbish existing space in the community and to equip the kitchen area with fridges, freezers, pressure cookers, and kitchen supplies. Food that was harvested was then brought into the centre where the women of the community would process it. Alongside, they would provide training for people wishing to learn how to prepare the animals and how to preserve them through canning, and drying or smoking (See Table 3.3 for food distribution details as documented by the community project lead). The centre also became a place where people came together for community cooking sessions. Led primarily by Rhoda Meekis and her daughter Arlene Jung, the sessions were designed to teach how to prepare healthy meals with the food harvested through the project. Traditional recipes were taught along with a variety of innovative ones—infusing local ingredients like wild rose petals into staple foods such as jelly and syrup, or using imported spices to make a sweet Thai chili with canned jackfish (northern pike). The positive and engaging environment Arlene and Rhoda created was formally recognized by the NAN; Arlene was awarded the Community Food Champion prize in 2012. Both Arlene and Rhoda are now highly sought after to perform cooking and food preservation workshops in the NAN region and they are truly leading in their efforts to build food sovereignty.

A second step that the community took to establish a sustainable food strategy was the development of family gardens. To construct a raised garden for each household, the residents utilized the knowledge Elders provided about traditional gardening in this area, and the northern gardening techniques Arlene experienced while living previously in Northern Manitoba. Funds from the project helped purchase frames and fencing materials, as well as enriched soils, plants, seedlings, and seeds. Project funds also paid shipping costs to bring these items into the community. Over the summer, all members of the community came together to help with the garden construction and maintenance and achieved what many did not know was possible in this region. In the first two years, primarily potatoes and onions were grown, but other items like lettuce and strawberries were also successfully planted. Each year innovative horticultural techniques are introduced and the gardens improve. Wawakapewin residents have also constructed

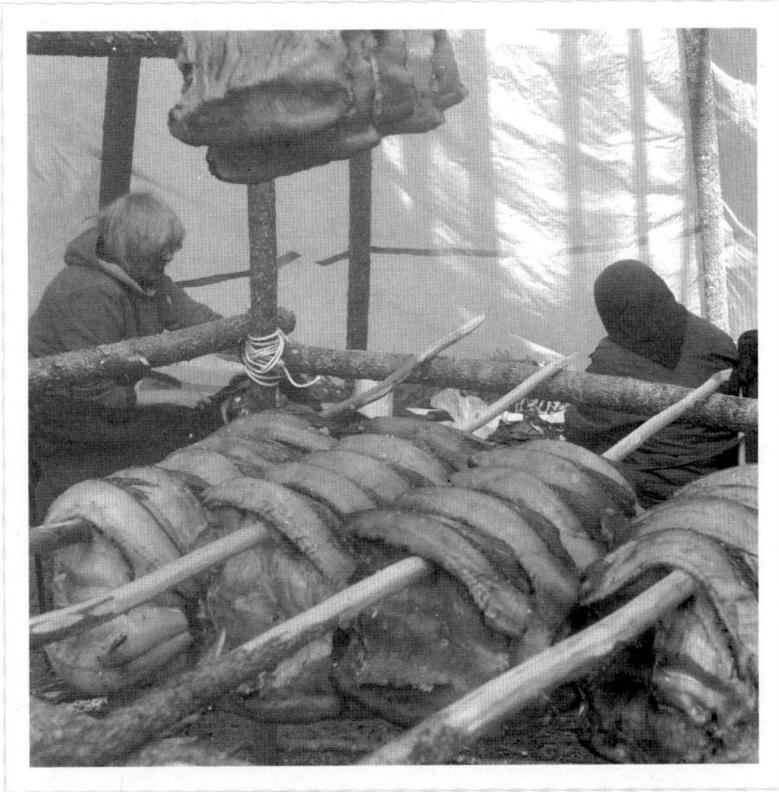

Figure 3.9. Inside a teepee at the Wawakapewin festival of Minookum, where land based teachings are taught, from teepee construction to food preservation.
Photograph by Courtney W. Mason.

a root cellar to help store what is harvested. This past winter, a makeshift greenhouse was constructed at the back of Arlene's house and in sub-forty temperatures, in January, tomatoes were growing. The gardens are a critical part of the overall Wawakapewin food strategy that thrives on local production and utilizes what the land provides.

Understanding the Impact of Community Food Projects

Over the course of this two-and-a-half-year funding period, the work demonstrated by each of these communities inspired us as researchers, but more so they inspired other Indigenous communities who sought involvement in

ACTIVITY	FOOD HARVEST AND/OR DISTRIBUTION
Downriver gathering 27 May–3 June 2011 Elders, helpers, children/ youth and staff ate wild food all week	About 40 fish netted each day (pickerel, whitefish, pike, and suckers) The men hunted with youth before the event to get beavers, geese, ducks 29 people ate wild food each day at the camp (fish, beaver, or ducks/geese) 2 meals per day, whatever was left over was distributed to the Elders to take home with them
Downriver gathering 27 May–3 June 2011 Distribution of smoked fish, beaver, ducks and geese	Each of the 9 Elders received 1.5 boxes of smoked fish, frozen fish, smoked beaver, and some ducks and geese (totalling 45 smoked fish, 9 ducks or geese, 18 frozen fish, and 3 beaver)
Sandy Point camp 26–30 September, 2011 Elders, helpers, children/ youth and staff ate wild food all week	About 50 fish in total, 1 beaver, 1 caribou, 6 geese 50 people in total, half of them children, were fed wild food every day (fish, beaver, or ducks/geese) 2 meals per day
Sandy Point camp 26–30 September 2011 Distribution of frozen ducks, geese, fish	Ducks (mallard, pintail) Canada geese, pickerel, whitefish Each of the 10 Elders received 1 box of smoked fish, frozen fish, smoked beaver, and some ducks and geese (totalling 40 smoked fish, 6 ducks/ geese, 18 frozen fish, and 2 beaver)
Sandy Point camp 30 September–5 October 2011	2 moose 15 community people remained at the camp distributing the 2 moose among their families and took the rest back to the community to distribute to community members (most of the meat was put in home freezers to last the winter)
Community garden September 2011	40 lbs of carrots; strawberries could not measure, as they were picked every day; lettuce provided for 4 homes each week, not measured

Table 3.3. Food Harvesting in the Wawakapewin First Nation.
Information in this table is a synthesis of the Wawakapewin First Nation community coordinator report highlighting program activities, costs and, outcomes over a six-month period.

the second phase of the project. CACO successfully secured two more years of funding, giving way to CACO II. In order to be eligible for the funding, our research team needed to demonstrate reach beyond the original jurisdictions in the first phase—therefore additional Indigenous partners needed to be involved. Part of the knowledge transfer component of the first phase ensured that our group and members from participating communities presented and co-presented at academic and public meetings and conferences, describing what they were doing. Hearing about this project, other communities began approaching our group asking if they too might be able to participate in this funding opportunity. Collaborative networks with other researchers, government personnel, and community organizations also grew as a result of the first phase of the project, providing ample opportunities for inter-jurisdictional growth and partnerships. At the time of writing the proposal, the challenge was not finding new community partnerships, but rather how to limit the number of partners and keep the project manageable, with the available time, funding, and personnel. In total, nine community partnerships were formalized for the grant proposal: three in the original Northern Ontario district, two in the Northwest Territories, two in Yukon Territory, and two in coastal communities of British Columbia.

The grant was based on the previous model whereby each community would develop their own plan to increase local food capacity. In CACO I, the original focus was on traditional food procurement, but as the project evolved, gardening became a valuable alternative. In this next phase, residents expressed interest in investigating more cost-effective ways of importing market foods into their communities and making fresh produce more readily available throughout the year. For example, in partnership with the Nishnawbe Aski Nation, a "Good Food Box" program was introduced into the Northern Ontario communities. This involved a wholesale company in Toronto and a food cooperative in Thunder Bay. By working outside of the Northern Store's for-profit food distribution model, individual families were able to order an extensive variety of fresh produce through the wholesale company and organize bulk transportation of food items with the assistance of the cooperative. The early stages of the program did enable families to receive high-quality food items at significantly lower prices, which led to more interest in the program and more families

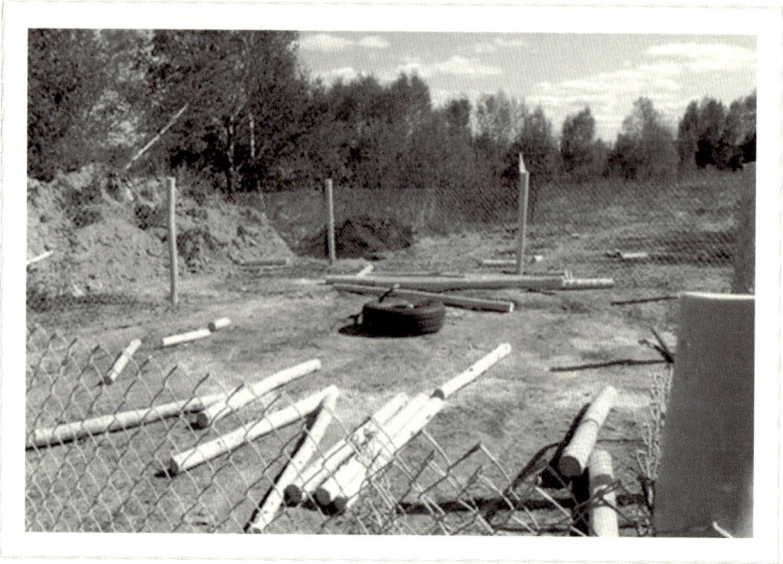

Figure 3.10. Early construction of the Wawakapewin First Nation community gardens. Photograph by Arlene Jung.

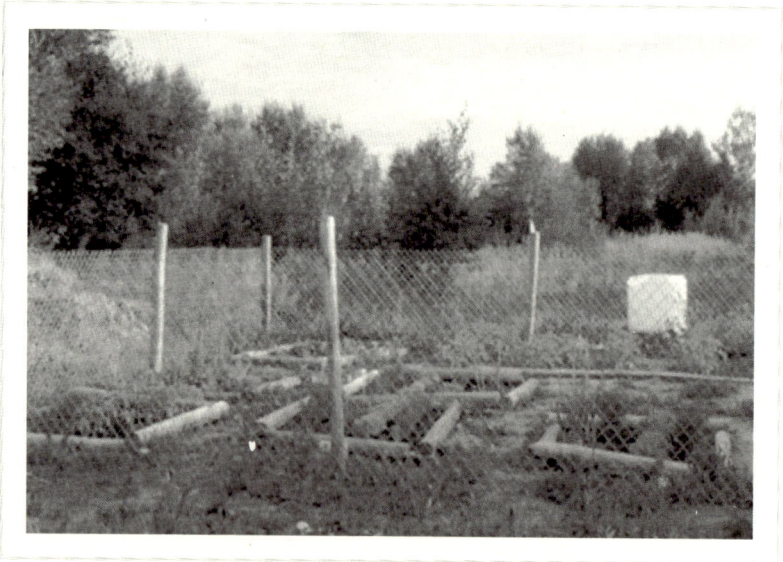

Figure 3.11. Wawakapewin First Nation community gardens by mid-point of the summer in year one. Photograph by Arlene Jung.

utilizing the service. However, there were challenges in running the program. In some cases, communities reported that the goods were frozen by the time they arrived and the produce was spoiled. In other cases, organizational issues within the communities made it difficult to get the food orders in, or distributed, once food arrived. The Nishnawbe Aski Nation is now working with communities to try to address these challenges, by learning where various breakdowns are occurring and by facilitating the ordering and distributing processes. The program, at the very least, suggests that there are affordable options for bringing healthy food items into these remote regions of the country—where profit-driven models fall significantly short and do not meet community needs.

As was the case in CACO I, the participating communities did demonstrate an improved capacity to harvest local foods, whether by gardening or by hunting and fishing. Local project coordinators were asked to record program activities and food yields. This provided information about the contributions of local food to the overall energy requirements per community. The coordinators' task was not easy with the amount and the variety of food that was being harvested. For example, people might go out and set nets and in some cases their catch would total over 100 fish. Measuring quantity, in terms of a number of fish, types of fish, and their weights, would have been ideal but was not realistic with the limited resources coordinators had at their disposal. Instead, estimates were provided whenever exact totals were not calculated. The coordinators also only reported on harvesting activities that were directly related to the CACO project; other harvesting did take place in the communities, but these yields were not estimated. Despite these limitations, we were able to gain some sense of the amounts and types of yields communities were able to procure as a result of the project. Based on the information that was provided, Indigenous Health Research Group members estimated total food harvests in terms of weight (when weight was not provided, average weights were used) and in total energy—broken down into proteins, carbohydrates, and lipids (fats). With this information, we were able to calculate each community's yield in relation to estimated energy requirements. In other words, working from the most basic individual energy requirements, we estimated the minimal amount of food a community needs in order to survive. This amount was

then compared with what food was harvested during the last six-month period of the CACO project to demonstrate how much locally produced foods
contribute to total energy requirements.

Despite the tremendous efforts and the considerable amount of food
produced through the project activities, locally produced foods make up a
mere fraction of the community's energy requirements. Figure 3.12 provides
a breakdown of one community's local harvest compared to what would be
required from the store in order to satisfy the minimum community energy
requirements. The information presented in this figure is representative of
the other participating communities. What is clear from this estimated data
is that local food efforts are producing significant yields, but these efforts
cannot be seen as the sole means of responding to the challenges communities face in acquiring regular access to healthy foods. These findings are not
meant to minimize the efforts communities are making to increase their
own local food production and procurement or the substantial yields each
community was able to produce or procure. Rather, they stress the need for
continued efforts and support in building local food capacity, which must
also include affordable importing and distribution of market foods.

Conclusion

The challenges northern Indigenous communities face in ensuring regular
access to affordable nutritious foods are multidimensional and extensive.
The efforts described in this chapter illustrate how some communities are
responding to these food challenges through local food procurement initiatives. The amount of food being produced, whether through traditional harvesting practices or through alternative means such as community gardens,
is considerable and will hopefully increase with the expansion of existing
programs. That being said, much more is needed to fully address northern
food insecurity and the subsequent health problems that these communities are enduring. Building local food procurement capacity is one approach
that is proving to be successful at various levels, but it is not close to meeting entire communities' food needs. Alongside these efforts, a strategy must
develop to reduce market food distribution costs and make nutritious foods
available and affordable in stores. There is a government program through
Nutrition North Canada that subsidizes the shipment of perishable food

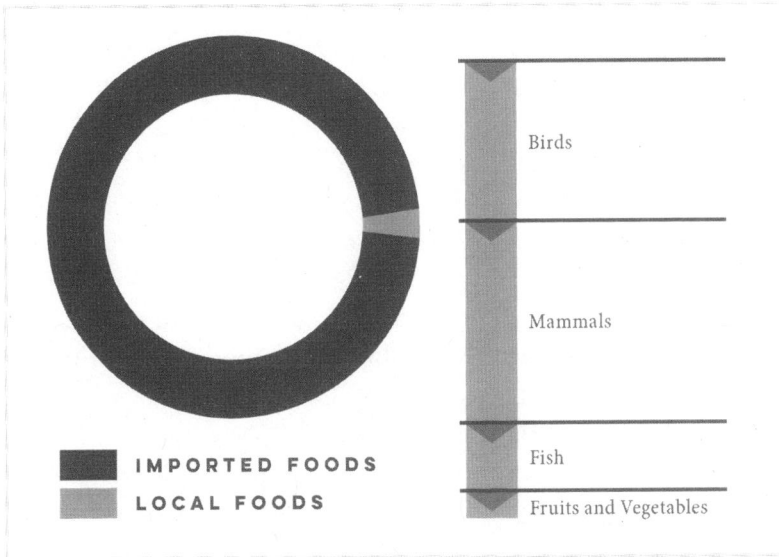

Figure 3.12. Estimated Contributions from Locally Procured Food Versus Market Food.

Locally harvested food represents 0.9 percent of total energy requirement of a remote
First Nation Community of Northwestern Ontario over a six-month period (April 2014–
September 2014). The contribution of locally harvested birds, mammals, fish as well as
grown fruits and vegetables (F and V) is also highlighted. Total energy requirement of
the community was calculated by assuming a total population of 485 members and a daily
energy requirement of 2000 kcal.

items to northern communities. However, the program has received notable
criticism. Many northern communities are not meeting the impractical
program eligibility requirements, and in other cases where subsidies are in
place, food prices remain high. The 2014 Auditor General's report revealed
that the program could not ensure that savings were being passed down to
consumers because retail prices were not being monitored. The report was
also critical of "unhealthy" food items being subsidized such as "ice cream,
bacon, and processed cheese spread" (Payton 2014, para. 7). Despite its limitations, the program does offer a necessary cost-saving mechanism that, if
more effectively implemented and enhanced, can have the desired impact of
making healthy food more affordable to northern residents.

Having access to healthy, affordable food is undoubtedly an important
first step in addressing food-related health concerns. In this chapter, our
group provides evidence of the significant increase in harvesting of local

food in various communities, and how these efforts are beginning to make healthy foods more readily available. However, we still need to assess how these efforts impact individual behaviours and if they lead to the positive changes necessary for chronic disease prevention or reduction. Are people eating healthier as a result of the local food initiatives operating in their community? If there are even slight improvements in diet, what impact are these modifications having on individual health? For us, as researchers working with communities toward addressing food-related health issues, the important next steps after developing and implementing initiatives will be to evaluate the effects these initiatives are having. Such data will provide important information about the overall value of these programs from the perspective of chronic disease prevention. If we can provide evidence that local food initiatives are positively affecting the health of individuals and communities, there will be greater likelihood of securing ongoing support. Researchers can play an important role by putting their findings into action and by helping communities maintain and develop local food initiatives in their efforts to improve community health.

Notes

1. Historically people in this region would consume all parts of animals to acquire essential vitamins and minerals, especially organ tissue, stomach content, bone marrow, and fats. While some people still eat various parts of the animal, it is predominantly muscle (protein) that is consumed (Robidoux, Haman, and Sethna 2009).

References

Anand, Sonia S., Salim Yusuf, Ruby Jacobs, A.D. Davis, Qilong Yi, H. Gerstein, P.A. Montague, and Eva Lonn. 2001. "Risk Factors, Atherosclerosis, and Cardiovascular Disease among Aboriginal People in Canada: The Study of Health Assessment and Risk Evaluation in Aboriginal Peoples (SHARE-AP)." *Lancet* 358 (9288): 1147–53.

Burnett, Kristin, Kelly Skinner, and Joseph LeBlanc. "From Food Mail to Nutrition North Canada: Reconsidering Federal Food Subsidy Programs for Northern Ontario." *Canadian Food Studies* 2 (1): 141–56.

Canadian Press. 2012. "Crisis Looming for First Nations Due to OxyContin." *CTV News*, 16 February. http://www.ctvnews.ca/crisis-looming-for-first-nations-due-to-oxycontin-1.769198#ixzz3CBcmgzM4.

CBC News. 2014. "Doctor Worried about Future of First Nations Addictions Program." 6 May. http://www.cbc.ca/news/canada/thunder-bay/doctor-worried-about-future-of-first-nations-addiction-program-1.2633869.

FNIGC (First Nations Information Governance Centre). 2012. *First Nations Regional Health Survey (RHS) 2008/10: National Report on Adults, Youth and Children Living in First Nations communities*. Ottawa: FNIGC.

Garrick, Rick. 2011. "Community Gardens a Hit in Remote First Nations." *Wawatay News*, 13 October. http://www.wawataynews.ca/home/community-gardens-hit-remote-first-nations. Haman, François, Benedicte Fontaine-Bisson, Malek Batal, Pascal Imbeault, Jules M. Blais, and Michael A. Robidoux. 2010. "Obesity and Type 2 Diabetes in Northern Canada's Remote First Nations Communities: The Dietary Dilemma." *International Journal of Obesity* 34 (1): S24–S31.

Imbeault, Pascal, François Haman, Jules M. Blais, Shinjini Pilon, Tim Seabert, Eva M. Krümmel, Michael A. Robidoux. 2011. "Obesity and Type 2 Diabetes Prevalence in Adults from Two Remote First Nations Communities in Northwestern Ontario, Canada." *Journal of Obesity* vol. 2011, 1–5.

Indian and Northern Affairs Canada. 2006. "Northern Food Basket." http://www.collectionscanada.gc.ca/webarchives/20071122024257/http://www.ainc-inac.gc.ca/ps/nap/air/fruijui/nfb/nfbont_e.html.

Kasabonika Fiscal Period 5 Report. 2012. April, unpublished community report.

NAN (Nishnawbe Aski Nation). 2012. "NAN Demands Response from Government on Opioid Epidemic and Anticipated Mass Withdrawal." News Release, 29 February. http://www.nan.on.ca/upload/documents/nr-feb-29-2012-nan-demands-response-from-governments-final.pdf.

Pal, Shinjini, François Haman, and Michael Robidoux. 2013. "The Costs of Local Food Procurement in Two Northern Indigenous Communities in Canada." *Food and Foodways* 21 (2): 132–52.

Payton, Laura. 2014. "Nutrition North's Impact on Northerners Uncertain, Auditor General Says." *CBC News*, 25 November. http://www.cbc.ca/news/canada/north/nutrition-north-s-impact-on-northerners-uncertain-auditor-general-says-1.2848653.

Robidoux, Michael, François Haman, and Christabelle Sethna. 2009. "The Relationship of the Burbot (Lota lota L.) to the Reintroduction of Off-the-Land Foods in the Sandy Lake First Nation Community." *Biodemography and Social Biology* 55 (1): 12–29. Willows, Noreen D. 2005. "Determinants of Healthy Eating in Aboriginal Peoples in Canada:

The Current State of Knowledge and Research Gaps." *Canadian Journal of Public Health* 96 (S3): S32–36.

Young, T. Kue, Jeff Reading, Brenda Elias, and John D. O'Neil. 2000. "Type 2 Diabetes Mellitus in Canada's First Nations: Status of an Epidemic in Progress." *Canadian Medical Association Journal* 163 (5): 561–66.

Chapter Four

TRAVERSING THE TERRAIN OF INDIGENOUS LAND-BASED EDUCATION

Connecting Theory to Program Implementation

As Chapter 1 demonstrates, the lifestyles of Indigenous peoples were drastically altered through government policies designed to dispossess them of their lands and resources, and to assimilate their cultures into the dominant Euro-Canadian model of the emerging Canadian nation state. Treaty agreements, the reserve system, and residential schools contained Indigenous communities and limited their abilities to pursue their subsistence and cultural practices. Without access to their lands and resources, Indigenous people could not engage in land-based activities. In Chapter 2, the authors indicate how these barriers had significant consequences for knowledge production, culture, and health in Indigenous communities across the country. First, this chapter will briefly overview how these historical changes disrupted the established lifestyles in regard to Indigenous methods of knowledge production. Then, shifting to a contemporary orientation, we will centre on how Indigenous knowledge systems can be reclaimed through the development of land-based educational programs and curriculum. We will draw on our own participation in land-based educational practices, to consider the challenges and possibilities of designing and implementing these programs in Indigenous communities. This chapter is based on semi-structured and unstructured interviews with Oji-Cree Elders. The interviews were conducted in the spring of 2011 while we participated in a food gathering festival known as Minookum. Briefly mentioned in Chapter

3, Minookum is described at length below. We also employed ethnographic methods in our fieldwork in one Oji-Cree community (Wawakapewin) in the Nishnawbe Aski region of Northwestern Ontario.

This chapter will address the following key questions: What are the historical factors that have distanced some communities from land-based educational practices? Why are land-based educational programs a productive way to learn for Indigenous communities? And, can communities reclaim their education by taking Indigenous-centred approaches of knowledge production from theory to practice? We contend that although there are significant historical and practical challenges to instituting land-based educational curriculum, the potential benefits and possibilities of these programs make them a worthy investment for both the Indigenous communities and the broader Canadian society.

Disrupting Land-Based Education in Indigenous Communities
Prior to discussing the history of residential schools and the impacts they had, it is imperative to establish what Indigenous educational processes were in place before the arrival of Europeans on the North American continent. While differing in structure to European approaches, learning in Indigenous communities was facilitated through strategies that evolved over centuries or millennia of practice. As Miller explains:

> North American Indigenous peoples, like all humans
> everywhere, possessed systems of education even though
> they did not have schools prior to the coming of Europeans.
> Like most successful pedagogical complexes, their
> educational approaches simultaneously reflected the values
> the adult community shared and instilled them in the next
> generation. The curriculum of this instruction told young
> people who they were, what other beings around them
> were, and how the humans and other beings related to one
> another. It explained where they all came from and where
> they were destined to go, what the dangers and opportunities
> of the journey were, and what obligations and rights, both
> individual and collective, they had. And it prepared them to

be successful mothers, providers, defenders, instructors, and
leaders of their own communities. (1996, 38)

Despite the common approach characterized above, it is also important to
emphasize that different Indigenous groups, individual bands, or communities applied diverse educational methods. As one might expect with varying economies and social and political structures, Indigenous groups across
the continent applied diverse pedagogical methods in their communities.
However, common among them were instructional processes that relied on
developing strong listening and observation skills (Barman, Hébert, and
McCaskill 1986). These skills were central to effective learning because children were taught while engaging in land-based practices. In this respect,
learning was integrated into the quotidian rhythms of life in the community
and travelling on the land. Whether it was through play, listening, watching,
or participating, the education of children was not partitioned off from other daily tasks. At first Europeans had difficulty understanding the lack of
structure in Indigenous education. As Oji-Cree Elder Simon Frogg explains:
"We Aboriginal people learn in a different way. It's not in a structured way
like some other people do. When we decide we want to do something, we
go out and do it. There's nothing structured or systematic about it . . . or
in the European way at least. I realize that it's different" (Frogg 2011, Personal interview). While there were most certainly structures and timetables
in Indigenous pedagogical strategies, ones that had come into place over
generations, they often contrasted European approaches and therefore were
misread or misinterpreted by European colonizers.

As discussed more thoroughly below, colonial influences on educational processes in communities have frequently fostered distrust of Euro-
Canadian political and education models. Archie Meekis, an Oji-Cree man
from Wawakapewin, discusses the general suspicion of government initiatives in many communities: "they think that the government is trying to or
is putting these programs in place to understand their way, their culture,
their traditions and their values and then that way they can get rid of them.
Seriously, that's what a lot of people think. When is that infected blanket
coming out again?" (Meekis 2011, Personal interview). Meekis's words explain why there exists what can be characterized as a perceived disinterest

among Indigenous peoples in institutionalized education over the latter half of the twentieth century. Oji-Cree Elder Jeremiah Nanokeesic elaborates further when discussing government educational institutions: "The education system itself is a problem or the way education has been set up. In our communities, as soon as a child entered education, that's when the process of leaving their culture and identity began. It was a different cultural influence that was being instilled in them. It was a process where they left their culture when they left being on the land" (Nanokeesic 2011, Personal interview, interpreted by S. Frogg). For many communities, particularly those impacted by residential schools, formalized European education has only recently become valued. This is especially the case in isolated rural regions of the country (Barman, Hébert, and McCaskill 1987). Drawing on the working experiences throughout his life, Nanokeesic emphasized how, in northern communities, men and women had to strategically educate themselves. They developed diverse skill sets to perform numerous tasks in the community, sometimes entirely without formal education. Here is part of Nanokeesic's discussion of his work and informal education:

> I am saying that for me, I'm sitting here and I can't
> communicate in the English language. I never went to
> school in my lifetime, but I did all the things that were
> asked of me to do without formal structured education.
> For example, the airstrip in Big Trout Lake . . . there were
> only two of us that constructed it. That airport is still in use
> today. The years I was in Big Trout Lake I handled all of the
> work involving machinery. I had to learn how to operate a
> sawmill and heavy machinery like tractors, bulldozers, or
> whatever. At a point in time, there was commercial fishing
> and there was a big inboard boat that I used to drive too.
> Also, I was a councillor for several years, then a chief for ten
> years, now I'm a minister. Why I'm saying this is that for
> me to do something, you can be educated in many different
> ways. I accomplished all this without being educated in
> the European way. (Nanokeesic 2011, Personal interview,
> interpreted by S. Frogg)

Despite the incredible accomplishments of Nanokeesic, formal and institutionalized education was not part of his training. The school systems, initiated by missionaries and the government, did not have the same influence in his community when he was young as they did in the late nineteenth century and they do now in the twenty-first century. In his discussions on this matter, it was clear that the presence of residential schools, or at least the community's negative response to their presence, produced a gap in structured learning in many Indigenous communities in Northwestern Ontario and across the rural North (Nanokeesic 2011, Personal interview interpreted by S. Frogg).

Another aspect that was considered widespread in most Indigenous educational approaches was the emphasis placed on listening. Similar to many cultures around the world, Indigenous peoples in Canada belonged primarily to oral cultures. Consequently, developing strong listening skills was a necessary component to lifelong learning. Every aspect of development, from practical tasks to spiritual growth, was facilitated at least partly through the sharing of narratives. As Miller notes, "stories . . . were used to transmit ethical, theological, historical, ecological and political information in societies in which almost no writing was available. It was through stories, for example, that children of all communities learned how their world came to be and where they fitted into it" (1996, 25). In her study of Indigenous histories of the Saint Elias Mountains of Northern North America, Cruikshank (2005) reveals that Elders and knowledgeable adults in the community would contribute to the education of all the children and that many of their lessons were facilitated through the telling of, and listening to, stories. In addition to teaching specific tasks and supporting cultural and linguistic continuities, narratives were constantly shared in processes designed to instill particular values, ethics, and corresponding behaviour. Before we highlight how residential schools produced a disruption in Indigenous systems of knowledge production and educational strategies, it is critical to provide a brief overview of how the schools developed throughout the country and how Indigenous peoples responded to these intrusions into their communities.

Histories of Residential Schools:
Colonial Intentions and Community Responses

As early as 1620, an order of Franciscans, known as the Récollets, established the first boarding school in Canada for Indigenous students. Despite the opening of other schools, many of the early residential school programs in New France failed because they did not correspond to European interests. Europeans needed Indigenous peoples to participate in the fur trade economy and in the various conflicts between competing European nations—both ventures requiring them to be mobile. However, beginning in the mid-nineteenth century, having Indigenous youth attend residential schools became a priority for the colonizers. As Indigenous peoples were no longer necessary fur-trade partners or military allies, they came to be primarily considered as barriers to progress and European settlement (Miller 1996).

Throughout much of the early history of residential schools, church leaders had a significant amount of control over the schools' operations. This made the schools more affordable for the government, as missionaries were much cheaper to hire than qualified teachers. In 1894, the government legislated compulsory attendance in residential schools, although it was not enforced in many communities. One year prior, in 1893, the government instituted a per capita system, which regrettably remained in place until the 1950s. This system produced a number of significant issues for administrators of the schools and ultimately for the pupils and their families (Haig-Brown 1988). Under the per capita system, levels of enrolment became more important than graduation rates and the quality of education. Missionaries aggressively recruited children from local and regional reserves to get government funding. When attendance levels were low, funding was cut and the quality of the living conditions plummeted, and this made recruiting children even more difficult. To address this issue, in 1920 the Indian Act was amended to make residential school attendance compulsory for all Indigenous children, age seven to fifteen (Miller 1996). In 1933, the government made further steps to enforce this legislation when it recruited members of the Royal Canadian Mounted Police (RCMP) to act as truant officers. Moreover, the 1945 Family Allowance Act required residential school attendance in order for families to have access to baby bonuses and other sources of subsistence. All of these measures were designed by the government to ensure that as many children as possible attended residential schools (Barman, Hébert, and McCaskill 1987).

While it is difficult to define the complex motives and objectives of various arms of government and of individuals participating in the colonial bureaucracy, legislation concerning the schools had a number of defining features and specific intentions. Guiding the decisions made by the colonial bureaucrats were a number of underlying assumptions about the racial superiority of Euro-Canadians compared to other new immigrants and Indigenous peoples. In the late nineteenth century, the government instituted several laws to limit specific immigrant groups from permanently taking up residency in Canada. These notions of the racial superiority, especially among Canadians of Western European descent, also informed policy regarding Indigenous peoples during this period. In his seminal history of residential schools in Canada, Miller (1996) convincingly argues that residential schools were primarily viewed as instruments to assimilate Indigenous peoples into the broader Canadian society during a period of incredible disruption and transition for most Indigenous communities. The Canadian government pursued opportunities to assimilate Indigenous children through residential schools precisely at a time when many communities were vulnerable and consumed with managing drastic changes to their lifestyles.

In the late 1920s, there were seventy-seven residential schools across the country and an additional 250 day schools for Indigenous children. At their highest attendance levels, 30 percent (6,641) of the potential 20,419 Indigenous children between the ages of seven and fifteen attended residential schools in Canada (Miller 1996).[1] In total, from the 1870s until 1996, it is estimated that over 150,000 Indigenous children attended the schools (Barman, Hébert, and McCaskill 1987). Despite the legislation and related efforts of the Canadian government to make residential schools compulsory, communities did not sit idly by. Many people took action when they disagreed with, and in some cases resented, the intrusion into their communities and the disruption of their lifestyles, especially through Euro-Canadian approaches to educating their children. One of the most common ways parents resisted residential schools was simply to refuse to have their children attend altogether or attend regularly (Haig-Brown 1988). There were also more visible forms of resistance, including confrontations between administrators or teachers and Indigenous parents and leaders. These altercations were often the result of community members trying to protect their children against unjust living conditions or, in some cases, forms of sexual and physical abuse. It is now clear that abuse was endemic in many schools across the country and this was regularly a source of conflict (Milloy 1999).

In addition to not sending their children to residential schools, communities also resisted the forms of cultural repression that the schools instituted or attempted to institute. The best example of resistance to the schools and their policies was the persistence of Indigenous linguistic and cultural practices. There were only a few residential schools where pupils did not experience severe forms of linguistic and cultural repression. To align with the government's broader legislative attempts to assimilate Indigenous peoples, the schools banned the use of Indigenous languages and forbade most cultural practices. As outlined in Chapter 1, legislation targeted practices such as the Sun Dance, the Potlatch, and the sweat lodge ceremonies, which were all made illegal in 1885 (Bracken 1997). In rare cases, in Manitoba and in James Bay, Ontario, the curriculum did attempt to integrate subsistence lifestyles of local peoples, but as a general rule Indigenous subsistence practices were discouraged and at times demonized. As early as 1880, the federal government pursued the policy referred to as the "bible and the plough." These measures were designed to assimilate Indigenous peoples so they would become Christian and would practise agriculture. Even though many North American climatic zones and ecosystems, where subsistence practices flourished for millennia, were not suitable for agricultural production, subsistence practices such as hunting, fishing, and gathering were viewed as highly problematic, by government officials and missionaries alike. The attempts to curb Indigenous subsistence practices had little to do with providing Indigenous people with a sustainable food source. Many communities across the country were healthy and were successfully providing local and regional food to their members for generations (Snow 2005). Curbing subsistence practices mainly supported broader assimilation strategies. For example, it did not suit the officials that families follow seasonal game and leave the reserve. If they were not living sedentary lifestyles in permanent communities, Indigenous people could not be exposed to assimilatory institutions such as churches and residential schools.

On many reserves throughout the country the dependency of communities on rations was not an inevitable sign of changing political and economic structures or environmental conditions, but a result of wider assimilation strategies (Mason 2014).

The divides that were created in Indigenous communities were perhaps some of the most damaging consequences of the cultural and linguistic repression in residential schools. Teaching students that their cultures and languages were primitive, pinned students against their relations in their communities. In preventing students from learning their culture—whether it was how to heat stones for a sweat lodge, how to process and preserve fish, or how to track large mammals—residential schools facilitated a knowledge gap in communities. Parents and grandparents of the students lived a more traditional lifestyle, but the students who lived away at the schools lacked the skill sets to do so. Additionally, their training at the schools sometimes demonized Indigenous languages and cultures, and some students began to resent these practices and their own families. These partitions within families grew when students returned home from years of training in residential schools and felt that they did not really belong in their own communities. At the same time, many of them lacked the skills to gain employment in urban centres and in many cases faced incredible discrimination and racism in broader Euro-Canadian society. By being displaced from their communities, students were critically affected in several ways. Parenting was one of the skill sets that students did not properly develop at residential schools. As they could not learn by engaging with and observing their own parents (missionaries and church staff were poor parental substitutes), students did not have access to these essential learning and growth experiences. This remains a great concern in some communities decades later. Miller explains, "students who had not learned how to relate to others in a familial setting grew into adults who often did not know how to act as parents. The lack of parenting skills has frequently been cited as a major problem affecting Native families and communities down to the present day. The breakdown of families that resulted in spousal and child abuse, desertion, alcoholism, and substance abuse has been a plague in Native communities" (1996, 339). It is clear that the residential school system was deleterious to families and communities on several levels. It disrupted the culturally specific transmission of knowledge and, under an assimilatory framework, introduced European ways of knowing.

Just the assimilation that took place in the schools was enough to brutally impact communities. As Miller (1996) writes, "It severed the ties that bound Native children to their families and their communities, leaving semi-assimilated young people and shattered communities" (10–11). Despite the assimilatory frameworks that guided almost all of the residential schools in the country, it is essential to recognize that Indigenous children and communities did refuse to assimilate and did express considerable resistance to the strategies designed to repress their cultural and subsistence practices (Haig-Brown 1988). Historians, anthropologists, and other scholars have often misinterpreted enrolment in residential schools or attendance of other European institutions, such as church, as being representative of the level of cultural assimilation reached in a community. However, there are active and passive forms of resistance. Indigenous peoples sometimes strategically engaged in Euro-Canadian institutions and also simultaneously pursued their own linguistic and cultural practices (Alfred 1995, 2009; Mason 2012). Their resistance to and dissent over the presence of residential schools in Indigenous communities was not limited to the first few decades of the twentieth century. Forms of resistance began to mount as the century progressed. After the Second World War, the protests by Indigenous and non-Indigenous groups in Canada forced the government to reconsider the residential school system. In 1946, a committee was created to assess what alternatives existed. Two years later, this committee presented Indigenous critiques of the system and called for more community-based controls of the schools. Even though the government refused to compromise and make the necessary changes, leaders in Indigenous communities began to organize their resistance against the schools. This was a key step that eventually led to the demise of the entire system. In the 1960s, Indigenous organizations, such as the National Indian Council and the National Indian Brotherhood, actively expressed their dissent concerning the schools and their impacts on communities. It was in the late 1960s climate of activism and assertion of human rights that Indigenous organizations found allies in non-Indigenous supporters. The general frustration of religious leaders and some government officials also contributed to the end of the misguided and dysfunctional educational system. In 1973, Indigenous political leaders, who themselves could speak first-hand about the issues in residential schools, led the charge, and the federal government relinquished its control of Indigenous educational systems (Barman, Hébert, and McCaskill 1987).

It was not until 1986 that religious authorities, led by the United Church of Canada, made public apologies for their roles in the residential school system. The federal government waited even longer to issue a public apology. In 1998, it finally released a Statement of Reconciliation, which also included an apology to the individuals who were abused in residential schools. At the same time, the Aboriginal Healing Foundation was formed to fund projects facilitating community-based healing. In 2005, the government announced a more comprehensive compensation package for victims of the school system. This also led to the 2006 Indian Residential Schools Settlement Agreement (IRSSA), the 2008 Truth and Reconciliation Commission of Canada (TRC), and the prime minister's public apology in front of the cabinet and Indigenous delegates. All of these initiatives were designed to recognize the problems that residential schools caused in Canadian Indigenous communities, to compensate students, and to provide support to those who suffered abuse at the schools. Despite these attempts to address some of the injustices permitted under the residential school system, healing has really only just begun in many communities across the country.

The TRC, which originated from the IRSSA, has significantly facilitated the beginning of this healing process. The Commission's work started in June 2008 and was completed in December 2015; it was a comprehensive response to the charges of abuse by former Indigenous students. The process involved a six-year investigation into the experiences of approximately 6,000 Indigenous students in residential schools. Of the approximately 150,000 children who attended the schools, many students suffered physical, mental, and sexual abuse. The Commission studied archival records, took testimony of what occurred at residential schools, and then issued a document identifying ninety-four calls to action. These calls not only meant to help redress the legacy of residential schools, but also to move the reconciliation process forward.[2] The report findings were divided into two relevant categories: legacy and reconciliation. To redress the harms of the Indian residential school system, the legacy section recommended increasing funding to improve child welfare and access to legal systems for Indigenous peoples, addressing inequities between non-Indigenous and Indigenous Canadians in education and health, and supporting education in Indigenous languages. The reconciliation part of the report centred on the Canadian government's lack of commitment to the United Nations Declaration on the Rights of Indigenous Peoples. It also singled out the support of youth programs and the redesigning of education as key aspects to meet the needs of Indigenous communities. In the context of our work, we outline the mental and physical health consequences of the schools that continue to impact Indigenous peoples.

Health Impacts and Enduring Legacies of Residential Schools
In addition to cultural loss and the disruption of families, health impacts of residential schools continue to influence educational processes in Indigenous communities. The physical, emotional, and sexual abuse of children did have and continues to have some of the most traumatic effects on Indigenous peoples, but there were also numerous other health concerns within the residential school system. Poor living conditions, starvation, and disease were some of the realities of day-to-day life that students endured in residential schools. In 1904, Dr. P.H. Bryce carried out an investigation into the health conditions of residential schools throughout the prairies. He was a medical officer for both the Interior Department and Indian Affairs and his findings were published. After extensive examination of the overall health of the schools, he recommended significant investments in health facilities to improve medical testing and general living conditions (Miller 1996). Since no measures were taken following his 1911 report, in 1922 he published a scathing account titled *The Story of a National Crime.* In it, he criticized the government officials and missionaries for failing to provide minimal health standards for students. His report provided ample evidence that children were suffering from neglect, poor nutrition, lack of warm clothing, and inadequate access to medical services (Milloy 1999). In reference to Bryce's report and the government's failure to address the basic needs of children, Miller surmises: "at times it was difficult to tell if the department's view that Aboriginal peoples were a 'dying race' was an observation, a prediction, or a policy assumption" (1996, 302). In addition

to deplorable health conditions at many schools across the country, Ian Mosby's research has revealed that some residential schools were also used as laboratories for biomedical science and experimentation. For a ten-year period, between 1942 and 1952, nutrition researchers worked in collaboration with various federal departments and missionaries to conduct a series of nutritional studies on Indigenous communities and residential school pupils in Northern Ontario. This work points to another level of misjudgment, exploitation, and neglect by the Canadian government in its treatment of Indigenous students in residential schools, as well as the schools' consequent health impacts for numerous generations (Mosby 2013).

An absence of adequate government funding was clearly a factor in the poor health conditions of most schools. Even the physical, sexual, and emotional abuse, which was a major issue at many institutions, can be linked to poor investment in the education system. There was constantly a shortage of trained and qualified staff in the schools. The formal training of teachers, administrators, and childcare and health care workers really only began in the late 1950s (Milloy 1999). Also the selection of staff members based on their religious training and not on their knowledge of education or health was problematic. In far too many cases staff members accused of abusing students were reassigned to another school in the system, instead of being criminally prosecuted. Because perpetrators were not held accountable or punished, a culture of abuse developed and thousands of students suffered in the schools. Despite the documentation of extensive and various forms of abuse, it is important to recognize that there were also compassionate, knowledgeable, and committed staff—working tirelessly for decades to provide the best education and care for students without appropriate recognition or compensation. It is for this reason that some students have had positive associations with residential schools and the people that cared for them (Barman, Hébert, and McCaskill 1986). Unfortunately, the overwhelming evidence of abuse, poor health, and sub-standard living conditions overshadows these positive experiences. It is now clear that many of the critical health issues could have been avoided if the staff were adequately paid and the institutions were properly funded. However, better quality education and higher health standards at the schools would have required a massive increase in the overall school budgets, and the government was unwilling to make these contributions (Barman, Hébert, and McCaskill 1986). As noted above, Indigenous organizations did not form a significant power block until the 1960s and Indigenous peoples could not vote until 1960. These had to be important factors in the government's decisions to ignore the repeated calls to improve social and health conditions at residential schools.

Understandably, as a remnant of residential schools, there remains a distrust of government health and educational institutions in many Indigenous communities. Across the country, communities have been left fractured and many people continue to heal from the reoccurring abuse they have experienced. Over the last decade, more residential school students have been finding the courage to report their physical, sexual, and emotional abuse, and for many this means reliving these horrendous experiences in detail. TRC findings indicate that the health issues related to the abuse have manifested themselves in generations of Indigenous peoples. While many communities have made significant strides in regaining their land-based subsistence practices as well as their cultural and linguistic knowledge, the schools created generational gaps that will forever impact how knowledge and culture is produced and transmitted in Indigenous communities. Therefore, in agreement with many leaders and educators, we contend that designing and implementing educational curriculum that engages students through participation in land-based practices is necessary. Such curriculum will foster Indigenous systems of knowledge production and cultural practices that were so vehemently targeted and repressed through the residential school system.

Reclaiming Education and Indigenous
Systems of Knowledge Production
As established in the previous section, Indigenous ways of knowing have been marginalized in Canada through assimilatory educational processes that served colonial interests. In addition to this historical context, it is critical to overview the contemporary scholarly literature on Indigenous systems of knowledge production. In preparation for our journey to Northwestern Ontario, in the winter of 2011, we began to examine the literature that pertained to Indigenous ways of learning. We assessed scholarly work on traditional land-based activities and methods of learning from the land,

and on Indigenous knowledge and pedagogy. Incredibly diverse and constantly evolving to suit localized needs, Indigenous knowledge has been described by Mi'kmaw scholar Marie Battiste as an intricate web of relationships. Battiste explains that as a web such knowledge works "within a specific ecological context; contains linguistic categories, rules, and relationships unique to each knowledge system; has localized content and meaning; has established customs with respect to acquiring and sharing of knowledge; and implies responsibility for possessing various kinds of knowledge" (2002, 14). Although we are working in Canada to create educational initiatives that are inclusive of Indigenous knowledge and pedagogy, our work is also greatly informed by the research of international scholars (Smith 1999; Hickling-Hudson and Ahlquist 2003; Kana'iaupuni 2005; Meyer 2008; Smith 2009).

Cajete (1994) contends that through their relationships formed in association with community, land, animals, and plants, Indigenous peoples learn about life. These relationships are central to Indigenous pedagogies. The holistic elements of traditional education encompass physical, cognitive, spiritual, and emotional facets of the learner (Kovacs 2009; Anuik, Battiste, and George 2010) and need to include practical and land-based learning environments for students. Educators who search for ways to teach holistically understand that connecting students to their spirituality is a distinct challenge (Curwen Doige 2003). As we will discuss, opportunities for students to develop physically, cognitively, but especially emotionally and spiritually can be nurtured while they are on the land, participating in community food-gathering activities such as the Wawakapewin First Nation's celebration of Minookum. Community members believe that through land-based education during Minookum, and similar annual food-gathering festivals, there is great potential to reclaim the production and transmission of Indigenous knowledge. Community Elder Simon Frogg is deeply committed to developing a land-based curriculum for the youth in his community. He states that: "We are starting to get back what we lost, we have been misled. You know we have allowed ourselves to be extracted from the main thing that has been given to us . . . and now we are trying to make an effort to gain back some of what we had" (Frogg 2011, Personal interview). Nanokeesic reinforces Frogg's point:

> Land-based activities can help us regain what we had in the
> past. This is an extremely difficult task because we lost so
> much of what we had in the past . . . we need to regain all the
> aspects of traditional knowledge, about the plants . . . planting
> the seeds and all that . . . it is also about the animals on the
> land, the fish in the water, the berries. I think it is proper
> that the government should be obligated to give us some
> resources so we can start to go back to regaining a part of our
> culture, our health, to exist in a way that is beneficial for us.
> (Nanokeesic 2011, Personal interview, interpreted by S. Frogg)

Despite the desire of community members to invest in land-based educational practices, there is little information on how to specifically develop a land-based curriculum to meet localized needs.

Redwing Saunders and Hill (2007) define the four domains that need to be considered in the development of practical land-based curriculum for Indigenous youth. These are holism, lifelong learning, community involvement, and authorship. Active participation in the daily activities of a community is integral to learning and education. Indigenous pedagogies consist of practical processes whereby students learn by watching, listening, and participating (Stiffarm 1998). Such learning can be fostered when students are connected to community and have access to hands-on experiences. In her discussion on critical pedagogy of place, Gruenewald (2003) asserts that student engagement can be attained through multidisciplinary, experiential, and intergenerational learning. Cajete (1994) argues that Indigenous education is in direct contrast to the prevailing education systems that emphasize objective content but are disconnected from community experiences. Historically, Indigenous youth received guidance through experience rather than through verbal instruction (Swan 1998). Battiste (2002) condenses Indigenous pedagogy into three interrelated components: observing, listening, and participating. The key to these methods is giving learners space and time to discover all three components and how they interrelate.

Since the land-based activities of Minookum depend on being on the land and experiencing fishing, hunting, and gathering of food, we turned to research that supported these aspects. In one recent study, Pearce and co-authors (2011) investigated traditional ecological knowledge and land skills among Inuit men in the Northwest Territories. They found that "land skills continue to be transmitted most often from older to younger genera-tions through observation and apprenticeship in the environment" (271). Their research indicated a high level of knowledge transmission and land-skill competence among these Inuit men. Perhaps even more importantly, their evidence demonstrated that there was simultaneous development of additional skill sets such as patience, observation, and control under pres-sure, as well as development of strategies to improve efficiency and execu-tion. While this research was conducted with young men aged eighteen and older, Pearce and colleagues did note that the local school had begun to facilitate fishing trips for their students to emulate the researchers' model, which centred on land-based experiences.

In a similar study, Takano (2005) investigated an Inuit land-based skills course where Elders took young men and women (aged seventeen to thirty-one) on the land. The study focussed on the diverse meanings being fostered by a connection to local lands, land-based practices, and intergenerational knowledge exchange. Takano observed that traditional ecological ways of learning were reinforced by allowing participants to repeat skills and to learn through trial and error. The emphasis was not on instant mastery or recall but on developing connections to their ancestors, local food gathering, and cultural sites, as well as the broader environment (Takano 2005). These con-nections were all facilitated through spending considerable time on the land with knowledgeable family and community members. Leighton Anderson from Wawakapewin emphasizes this when discussing Minookum as land-based education: "Being in places like this is how we bond with each other as there is a coming together of cultures and people that isn't the same on the reserve. This is how we understand our Elders and where and what we came from as Oji-Cree people. Our language, the way we treat each other or inter-act, the stories, the lessons or values in the stories only really make complete sense here. Without the land and us on it, all would be lost" (Anderson 2011, Personal interview). In their study that examined the transmission of inter-generational knowledge in Cree First Nations communities on James Bay, Ohmagari and Berkes (1997) also found that vital connections were made on the land among community members. The programs they evaluated were centred on female participants in land-based education. These studies (Ohmagari and Berkes 1997; Takano 2005; Pearce et al. 2011) all indicate that initiatives designed to learn from the land and to develop tangible skills through close guidance by knowledgeable community members were not historically encouraged by provincial and territorial educational systems in Canada. Also supported by evidence presented in Chapter 5, the above research suggests that land-based education fosters a strong connection between the land and community members, and this connection links participants to their linguistic and cultural practices. Despite their obvious benefits for Indigenous youth and communities, land-based programs are often marginalized in the existing institutionalized curriculum.

Prior to attending Minookum, we contemplated what kinds of opportunities and experiences students would gain by being on the land and learning from Elders and community members. Partly based on the above studies, we envisioned a curriculum centred on Indigenous pedagogies and knowledge that was entirely land-based. We recognized that land-based programs could empower students and instill a deep sense of connection to local cultural practices, community members, and regional ecosystems. Notwithstanding the compelling body of research, very few of these studies actually provided the specifics of land-based programs in relation to common Euro-Canadian models. This was critical because these prevailing systems of knowledge have, at least, overshadowed, and often completely marginalized Indigenous land-based approaches to education. However, it was unclear from the existing scholarship how these programs operate on the ground and how land-based curriculum practically contributes to reclaiming Indigenous systems of knowledge production. Understanding how the two systems, the Indigenous land-based approach and the prevailing Euro-Canadian model, have historically been facilitated in communities, and how they function in a contemporary context, is integral to developing new methods of land-based curriculum that meet localized community needs. Before we provide a map for developing a land-based Indigenous curriculum, we present our personal experiences of participating in land-based programs, to explain how our perspectives on these issues were formed.

Land as an Educational Resource: Personal Narratives of Minookum
COURTNEY MASON — In the spring of 2012, during the various flights travelling to Northwestern Ontario from the Southeast, I had sufficient time to consider the community-based research projects that I was now participating in as part of the Indigenous Health Research Group.[3] Puddle-jumping flights across a vast landscape of seemingly endless lakes and rivers provided opportunities for reflection. Because I grew up connected to local Mohawk communities in rural Eastern Ontario and this greatly impacted my own educational path, I was sensitive to how protective community members could be of reserve lands and spaces. Following five years of work with Nakoda peoples in Alberta throughout my doctoral studies, I was keenly aware of some of the power dynamics of working as an outsider in Indigenous communities. In Alberta, I was researching how the displacement from the Rocky Mountain National Parks, and the related policies to curb Indigenous subsistence practices, impacted health in Nakoda communities. In part, by using residential schools, the colonial bureaucracy took control of education away from local community members. Now travelling by air, the geography of Northern Ontario only seemed to emphasize the dissimilarities between Oji-Cree cultures and the Nakoda peoples whom I worked with in the foothills of the Rocky Mountains, but I wondered about their common colonial experiences. Even though my first trip to Oji-Cree communities presented new challenges under very different cultural contexts, I was interested to find out how similar colonial policies historically influenced these communities.

By the end of May 2011, I had already been working for one month at Kasabonika Lake First Nation. Then I flew back to Sioux Lookout to meet up with Desirée and, together, we set off for a traditional campground near Wawakapewin First Nation. In Oji-Cree, Wawakapewin means meandering river. Without an airstrip, the small community appeared more remote and isolated than others I had visited in the Nishnawbe Aski region. We were invited to participate in Minookum to learn about local food procurement and land-based education in Wawakapewin. Minookum is a traditional gathering held in some Oji-Cree communities; on the occasion community members assemble for educational, cultural, and food-procurement

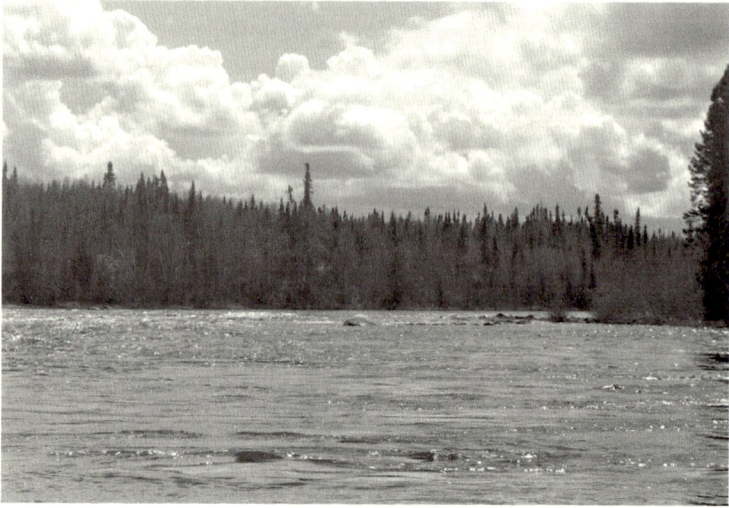

Figure 4.1. Remote location on the Ashewieg River system, between Wawakapewin and the community campsite for Minookum. Photograph by Courtney W. Mason.

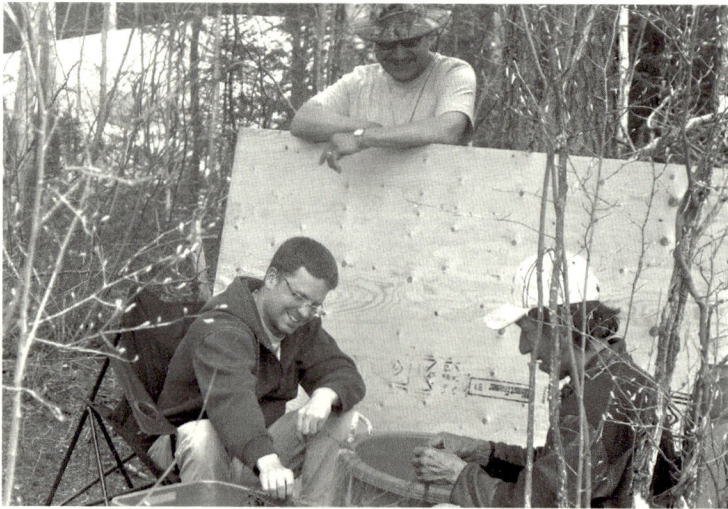

Figure 4.2. Mending the fishing nets. Co-author Courtney W. Mason (left) with community members Archie Meekis (above) and Leighton Anderson (right). Photograph by Desirée Streit.

activities. Desirée and I both felt honoured to participate in such an intimate cultural gathering.

After flying into a remote location along the Ashewieg (place of wait-
ing) River system, we met the thirty participating community members
and began to prepare the shoreline campsite. Incredibly, five generations
were in attendance at the camp. At first, many community members expressed interest in Desirée and me, but as could be expected, others seemed
a bit reserved with strangers in their community. Over the forthcoming
week, the tight-knit group seemed to accept and, at times, appreciate our
presence and contribution to the gathering. Over the next eight days we
were busy from early morning until mid-evening, every day. Men's activities were centred on building temporary camp structures for gatherings, as
well as for processing and smoking food. Hunting of primarily muskrat,
beaver, moose, and waterfowl were other key tasks. The men also fished
for northern pike, pickerel, whitefish, sturgeon, and red and white suckers. As discussed at length in Chapter 5, women focussed their efforts on
processing, cooking, and preserving food. Collecting plants and preparing
the communal spaces at the camp were other time-consuming jobs mostly
undertaken by women. We were told that during Minookum enough food
is often collected, processed, and preserved to meet the community's needs
for several months of subsistence.

When the weather permitted, community members were either out
on the water or busy in the camp. The activities were both physically and
mentally demanding. All community members shared in the work and
gathered to have collective meals. Eating and talking about food was a
central component of the experience and clearly one of the focal points
of the gathering. On the days when the weather was not as accommodat-
ing, people would gather in the teepees to visit and discuss various community initiatives. In informal land-use planning sessions individuals
brought up the distinct changes that their community was facing in the
immediate future (including natural resource development). They also
outlined and scrutinized various land-based educational initiatives meant
to encourage cultural and linguistic continuities. Desirée and I were there
to learn and welcomed our time working on the land with community
members and participating in the teepee sessions, which provided critical

socio-economic and cultural context for the community and the contemporary challenges that they were encountering.

DESIRÉE STREIT — Even before moving across the landscapes of Southeastern Ontario to the Northwest of the province, I prepared to embark on this research project by focussing on what my goals should be during my time with the Wawakapewin community on the land. After overcoming the excitement of being invited as an education researcher to participate in this unique experience, it was crucial for me to thoroughly think through how I should approach this project. My previous experience of working with Indigenous youth in after-school programs in urban Winnipeg was part of the research during my undergraduate degree in physical education. It taught me the importance of creating relationships when working with communities. Therefore, I was mindful that I was coming into this project with no connection to the community, and I wanted to be as sensitive and respectful as possible in the little time I had to establish a relationship with community members.

Even though I did not have a direct connection with the Wawakapewin community beforehand, upon arrival I felt an inherent bond, as I too come from a small northern community and I am an Indigenous woman. Growing up I did not identify myself as an Indigenous person even though I knew of my mother's heritage. At a very young age, she was removed from her community and placed with a Euro-Canadian family in the small northern town of The Pas, Manitoba. My mother's connection to her family and identity was severed when she was placed with this new family. Finding the way back to my Métis and Ojibwe roots did not begin until I was an adult. My journey steered me toward working with Indigenous youth, and this work, in turn, created a desire to take the steps to discover my heritage. Not knowing where to begin, I completed a minor in Native Studies at the University of Manitoba. During Minookum, to have the confidence to locate myself (Kovach 2009) as an Indigenous woman, in an academic and in a personal setting, was very empowering.

In order to maintain a respectful approach to the project in Wawakapewin, I wanted to refrain from thinking only as an education researcher. To shift my thinking, I set aside my Master's in Education. I wanted to step out of my role as a researcher and intentionally position myself as the learner instead. My goal for this trip was to experience what it meant to be on the land as a student or a beginner—going on the land for the first time with her community members. I felt that this repositioning would help me stay away from the temptation to judge or report experiences in such a way as to make them appear more educational. I thought that it was imperative to be open to the possibilities of being on the land, observing, listening, and participating in the activities and experiences of Minookum.

Allowing the experience to unfold consisted of letting go of what I thought the experience would be like, or what I thought the project would turn out to be. What I did not anticipate about this process was the amount of personal reflection on my past educational experiences that it would generate. It began as I moved across the changing landscapes—the shifting of hills to flatter skylines dominated by black spruce. Perhaps it was the spring air that produced these emotions, but as I travelled northwest I began to anticipate the topographic changes that I would see. I now reside in Ottawa, a part of Canada that I am unfamiliar with; there are trees that I do not know and lakes and skylines that are different from Northern Manitoba, where I grew up. As we journeyed to this remote community, only accessible by air, the feeling of coming home grew. The sensation of coming home also made me think of the Indigenous students that I was currently working with at a local high school in Ottawa. Many of them have to attend high school away from their home communities for various reasons. I recalled the excitement and joy they expressed when talking about going home to their communities and families in the northern parts of the province.

Even a year after our time in Wawakapewin, I continue to process the experience of being on the land with community members and Elders. What I experienced continues to enrich my life, inspiring and motivating me on many levels. Writing this excerpt with the objective of emphasizing the possibilities of land-based programs feels like a solidifying act, but what I learned is still with me, living and evolving the more I reflect on the experiences. There are so many moments that capture what it means to be on the land with people, in a social community setting. In each of these moments, there were opportunities to experience and witness how the production of Indigenous knowledge occurs at a localized level. There are two significant moments that I would like to discuss because they were used as a basis for creating the curriculum document that is presented below. The first occurred out on the water while setting fishing nets and collecting fish, and the second while filleting fish in the teepee with Elders and community members.

The feeling of camp was very welcoming and the location was beautiful. We were near the water, a strip of sandy beach, and a sheltered area for the cooking tent, communal teepee, and personal tents. The forest floor was covered with moss, making the ground comfortable to sleep on. Away from the water, the heat of the sun and lack of wind allowed for the Labrador tea that grew in the moss to release its sweet fragrance. All of these elements made the first day of being on the land very enjoyable, the kind of first day that sets the stage for the rest of the experience. My first impressions of being on the land were strengthened by the first time I headed out onto the water. Courtney and I were invited to set the nets on a calm, slightly overcast evening. Once again I began to feel nostalgia and my mind wandered back to all the boat rides I had taken with my own father at home in Manitoba. The liberating feeling of being on the open water is something I have always enjoyed. As we rode to the spot where we would set the nets, I was mesmerized by the mirror-like quality of the water that evening. The water reflected the overcast sky and it was hard to see where one began and the other ended except for the treeline, which was a dazzling mirror image of itself. The boat disrupted the water as we rode, creating beautiful ripples, and the fresh spring air opened up my lungs and the feeling of waking up from a winter sleep returned once again.

I was not sure what setting fishing nets entailed as I had only previously gone fishing with a rod and reel. I watched tentatively as Simeon Cutfeet, one of the two community members who took us out on the boat, carefully and skillfully set out the net. We watched as he adeptly untangled the net and set it down into the water without any twists or knots. He explained to us that we were putting the net where one river flows into the next, a good spot especially to catch whitefish. The long net was laid into the water, with weights keeping it in place at the bottom and floats at the top—these bobbed just above the surface. The following morning, we set out again to collect the fish, where we had set the net the previous night. The morning fog was lifting from the water and hovering on the shore, and the sun was peeking up over the trees. As we approached the net we could see there were indeed

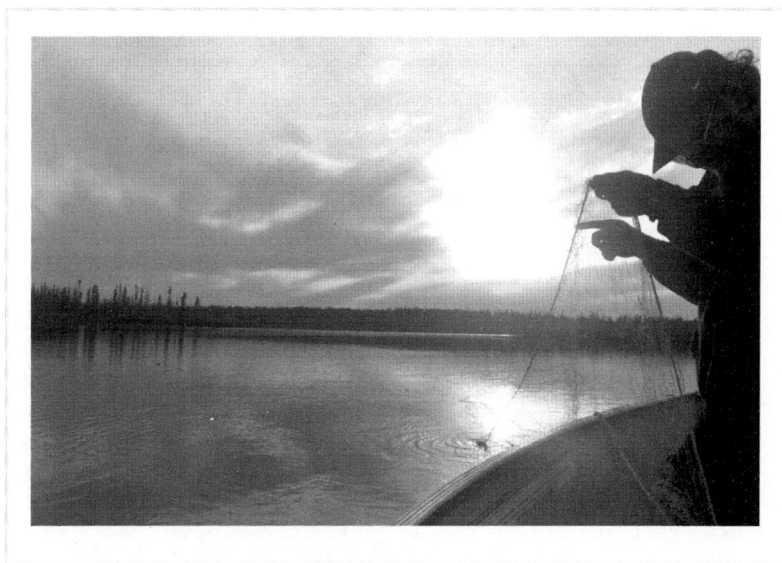

Figure 4.3. Community member Simeon Cutfeet setting fishing nets.
Photograph by Courtney W. Mason.

fish caught in it. Beginning at one end of the net, Simeon began the task of pulling up the net. As the net came out of the water, it was placed in a nearby bin. When Simeon reached a part of the net with a fish, he capably dislodged the fish from the tangled net, placed it in another large bin, and kept pulling up the net. The tool he used was a simple nail that had been bent into a U shape. It allowed him to pull the fine netting off from the body of the fish.

The second experience that stands out to me is an interaction I had with an Elder in the teepee used for filleting and smoking fish. I had spent some time in the teepee the previous day learning how to fillet whitefish, which are used to make pemmican. I remember being nervous about making mistakes, but with encouragement and the fact that there were so many fish to fillet, I soon became less anxious and enjoyed the learning experience. The following day I found myself wandering around camp before lunch. I decided to check out the teepee and see if I could lend a hand. It was a chilly day, so the teepee was a refuge from the cold. As I stepped through the door, my senses met the smoke from the burning coals, which rose up toward the opening at the top of the teepee. There was a mix of smells consisting of raw and cooking fish, duck, and beaver. Inside, I found an Elder sitting on the teepee floor covered in balsam branches. She was alone quietly filleting fish. I decided to sit with her and try my hand at filleting again. She made it seem effortless—scraping the scales off first with smooth swift strokes of the blade, she easily guided the knife to make precision cuts into the fish. I continued to watch the steps she took, before I got to work on the fish I was holding. My hesitation caught her attention and she gave me a quick smile. Using only gestures, because I did not speak Oji-Cree nor was her English very strong, she gave me a review by placing the knife where I should make the cuts. The exchange was brief but very effective. She watched as I took hold of the fish again and as I began to fillet, she laughed as if to reassure my efforts. I felt more and more competent in my ability to fillet as we worked together in almost complete silence.

Designing and Implementing Indigenous Land-Based Educational Programs

Once we returned to Ottawa, we had time to reflect on our experiences and could then turn our attention to creating a curriculum document appropriate for a land-based initiative, such as Minookum. We were inspired by the vision that Simon Frogg and other leaders of the community had for their youth. This vision centred on developing their connection to the land and to work within the curriculum framework of the province. In the initial stages of creating this document, we struggled with letting go of our own educational background dominated by Eurocentric values. We needed to honour the experiences of being on the land at Minookum and, importantly, not alter their character to fit provincial curriculum standards. The task involved examining Ontario curriculum to determine how it could support land-based experiences. We began by reading the Ontario curriculum for various grade levels, to assess how it could support land-based programs and localized needs. After detailed analysis, we chose to create a document centred on the grade six level (average age eleven). This was done for two specific reasons. First, in many remote regions students stay in their communities until this age, and in grade seven they move to larger centres to access further education, often in the South. As a result, the curriculum is designed to be of use in northern communities while students live locally.

Second, it was determined that this was an important transition or bridging year, whereby curriculum lessons could be adapted or modified to meet the needs of both younger and older students.[4]

In order to build this curriculum document, we needed to step back into the roles of educational researchers and focus on what the literature was suggesting about land-based initiatives and Indigenous pedagogies. Our curriculum document was designed to reflect Indigenous ways of knowing and learning, but a distinct component for the development of Indigenous languages was missing. Language is of course central to Indigenous cultures, especially in its transmission of important cultural knowledge (Pearce et al. 2011). Although we both have a basic understanding of Oji-Cree linguistic structure and vocabulary, our lack of linguistic competency was certainly a limitation in applying the program directly to local or regional contexts. However, we were assured by community members and Elders that this fundamental structure could be easily adapted to suit localized cultural and linguistic practices. This was in fact our intention from the beginning. It was evident from several experiences at Minookum that language components could easily be built into the curriculum structure. Below, we include excerpts from the curriculum document that we produced. It was designed as a guide for educators—to implement lesson plans that expand upon student experiences of Minookum or other land-based practices, and to also meet or respond to some of the expectations of provincial or territorial curriculums.

As established above and emphasized throughout this book, Indigenous ways of knowing and learning are closely connected to the land. Therefore, connections to land and place are integral to the development of Indigenous identities, confidence, self-esteem, pride, respect, and responsibility (Gruenewald 2003).[5] Through land-based activities, youth strengthen their web of relationships with local ecosystems, cultural practices, and community members. While each learner creates meaning from his or her experiences, the practices, lessons, and activities in this guide are meant to help students to reflect upon, explore, and apply the knowledge they gain from land-based programs to their own lives. Moreover, this guide has been developed with the intention of promoting a lifelong learning.[6] By harnessing a strong connection to the land through participating in activities, for example

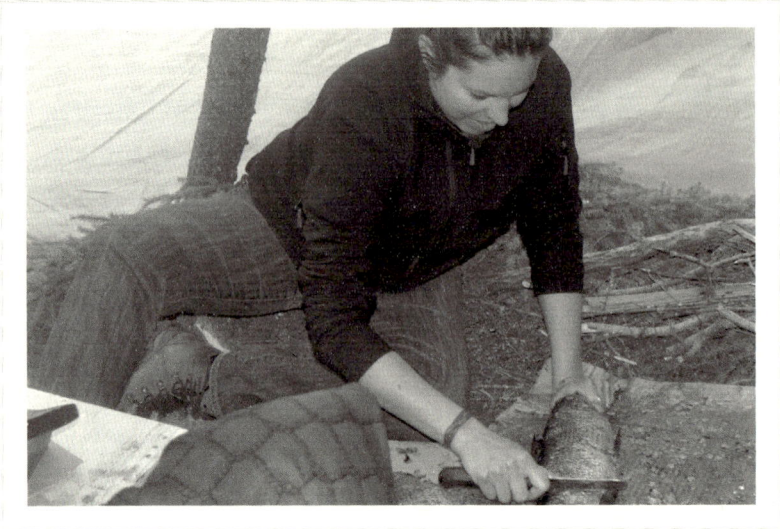

Figure 4.4. Co-author Desirée Streit learning from Elders how to descale white suckers. Photograph by Courtney W. Mason.

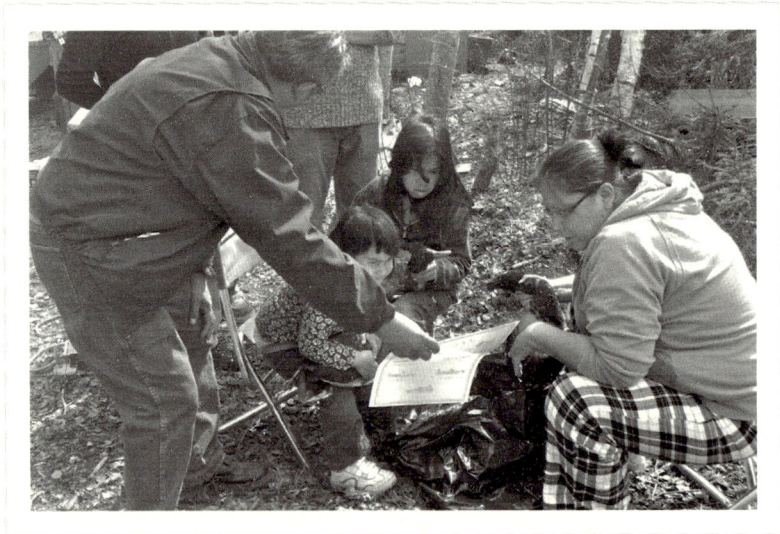

Figure 4.5. Community leader and Elder Simon Frogg teaches youth the Oji-Cree names for waterfowl found in the region and emphasizes their cultural importance as a local food resource. Photograph by Desirée Streit.

at Minookum, this curriculum aims to engage students in their education and support land-based knowledge and corresponding skill sets. In addition, this curriculum honours the concept of a holistic learner by incorporating the physical, cognitive, spiritual, and emotional elements of students' growth and experience. Central to this holistic approach is what Takano (2005) describes as a common sense of well-being—including health, happiness, pleasure, freedom, beauty, and quietness. Holistic approaches nurture opportunities where students can create positive connections to their community, their culture, and their identity, and we adapted this to specifically speak to participating in land-based activities. According to Kovacs (2009) and Anuik, Battiste, and George (2010), there are a number of holistic aspects to how students learn through land-based approaches. Within a holistic framework, learning also promotes self-awareness of the interconnectedness of diverse aspects of influence. As the scholars above contend, in many structured classroom settings physical and cognitive components of learning become the focus while spiritual and emotional elements are neglected. Being on the land and participating in land-based practices can help cultivate these areas, in individual and group learning sessions.

Purpose and Objectives Excerpted from the Land-Based Curriculum
The purpose of this curriculum guide is to engage Indigenous students in hands-on, practical, land-based education that fosters connections to local ecosystems and to community members while supporting cultural and linguistic continuities.

Objectives:

To promote learning and transmission of linguistic and cultural knowledge through hunting, fishing, and gathering activities on the land

To cultivate an appreciation for local food sources and systems, and traditional ways of cooking and preserving foods while promoting healthy nutritional choices

To develop a strong sense of connection to the land which will in turn facilitate relationships to local ecosystems, community members, and cultural values

To build confidence and motivation through land-based practices and cultural knowledge

Indigenous Pedagogies

The model used in this curriculum guide emphasizes some of the unique ways Indigenous cultures encourage learning and growth in their communities. As discussed above, Indigenous people historically learned on the land through observing, listening, and participating in family and community activities. As both Battiste (2002) and Takano (2005) argue, in this model instant mastering and recalling of skills are not expected. Instead, patience when learning new skills is emphasized. Through land-based activities, similar to those experienced during Minookum, students are encouraged to observe, listen, and participate in hunting, fishing, and gathering activities. For the most part, observation and listening are not accompanied with intervention or direct instruction, and participants are invited to engage only when they personally feel prepared and motivated. By reinforcing this way of knowing and learning, it is anticipated that students will learn from the experiences of being on the land and bring these methods to a classroom setting and apply them appropriately. The lesson plans in this curriculum document offer guidance to educators to help prepare students for their time on the land, and to facilitate purposeful reflection through activities and questions when they return to more structured class environments.

Using the Curriculum Guide

At the heart of this curriculum guide are the practical experiences of the students engaging in land-based practices. This model offers educational strategies for students, ones that place them in the curriculum as active players and not solely as recipients of information (Redwing Saunders and Hill 2007). Minookum itself is not being manipulated or altered in order to create learning experiences. Rather, the resources found in this document are designed to support the learning that occurs during Minookum. There

GOALS AND LEARNING OBJECTIVES

Through hands-on experience students will:

• Practise skills and learn the methods needed to net, process, and prepare fish during Minookum

• Gain a sense of connection to the land, themselves, and their community by observing, listening, and participating in traditional ways of preparing fish

By reflecting on their experiences connected to the land students will:

• Maintain a connection to important land-based experiences that will help inform their education/classroom learning

• Bring relevant experiences into the classroom as a resource to learn through cross-curricular activities such as healthy eating and living; science and technology; and language arts

PURPOSE/RATIONALE

The purpose of focussing on processing fish is to connect students to the traditional ways of gathering food on the land. Through this experience, students will gain practical knowledge of how to process fish, as well as develop personal attributes such as patience, cooperation, collaboration, and generosity.

TEACHER PREPARATION (RESEARCH, ORGANIZATION)

Preparation: background on what kinds of fish are caught, images of a variety of fish, how fish are prepared (traditional and current ways of cooking fish)

Example: Fish identification chart (Ontario)

MATERIALS/RESOURCES

• Text and images to support prior knowledge acquisition

• Flip chart and variety of coloured markers

• Journals

UNIT OUTLINE

Lesson 1: Preparing—Prior knowledge chart and journal preparation

Lesson 2: Response to journal and discussion

Lesson 3: Experiencing life on the land, Minookum video collage

Lesson 4: Creating public service announcement for healthy eating; Emphasizing why traditional food is important to Indigenous peoples

ASSESSMENT

• This unit can be assessed using students' journals, the completion of each of the following: "what I want to know chart"; Observing-listening-participation chart; Public service announcement graphic organizer; Storyboard

• The two video projects will also be included in the assessment: Minookum video collage and public service announcement

• Create rubric with students; Define what the criteria should be to assess their projects; Self-assessment and the creation of a learning rubric should also be incorporated into the evaluation

Figure 4.6. Example Unit Plan: Fishing. Source: Ontario, Ministry of Education, *The Ontario Curriculum: Elementary Grade 6*, 2010.

MINOOKUM (ON LAND)	REFLECTION AND CONTEXTUALIZATION (IN EDUCATION SETTING)

HEALTH AND PHYSICAL EDUCATION:

C. Healthy Living

C2: Making Healthy Choices
    C2.1 *Influences on healthy eating*
    C2.2 *Eating cues and guidelines*
    C2.3 *Safe and positive social interactions, conflict management*

C3: Making Connections for Healthy Living
    C3.1 *Benefits of healthy eating/active living*
    C3.2 *Responsibilities, risks–care for self and others, safety practices*

LANGUAGE:

Reading:
    1. Reflecting on reading skills and strategies (4.2 Interconnected skills)

Writing:
    1. Developing and organizing content
    2. Using knowledge of form and style in writing
    3. Applying knowledge of language conventions and presenting written work effectively
    4. Reflecting on writing skills and strategies

Media Literacy:
    3. Creating media text (3.1 Purpose and audience; 3.2 Form; 3.4 Producing media texts)

LANGUAGE:

Oral Communication:
    1. Listening to understand (1.1 purpose)
    2. Speaking to communicate (2.7 visual aids)
    3. Reflect on oral communication skills and strategies

SOCIAL STUDIES:

Heritage and Citizenship exemplar:

The task description specific to Grade 6 curriculum – identify one present-day concern of an Indigenous community related to how changes resulting from European contact affected the lifestyles of community members

    2. Describe the complex relationships between Indigenous peoples and their environments.
    7. Identify pressing concerns of Indigenous peoples.

    NOTE: At the time of print the social studies curriculum was revised from its 2011 version

NATIVE LANGUAGES:

Oral Communication – *Students should have many opportunities to listen to the Native language before they attempt to use the language to communicate.*

Overall Expectations – *Demonstrate knowledge and understanding of aspects of the Native culture under study.*

ARTS:

D. Visual Arts
    D1. *Creating and presenting (D1.1, D1.2, D1.3, D1.4)*
    D2. *Reflecting, responding, and analyzing (D2.4)*

MINOOKUM (ON LAND)	REFLECTION AND CONTEXTUALIZATION (IN EDUCATION SETTING)

SCIENCE AND TECHNOLOGY - BIODIVERSITY:

2. Developing Investigation and Communication Skills.

2.1 Follow established safety procedures for outdoor activities and field work (*e.g., stay with a partner when exploring habitats; wash hands after exploring a habitat*).

2.5 Use a variety of forms (e.g., oral, written, graphic, multimedia) to communicate with different audiences and for a variety of purposes (*e.g., use a graphic organizer to show comparisons between organisms in various communities*).

3. Understanding Basic Concepts.

3.1 Identify and describe the distinguishing characteristics of different groups of plants and animals (e.g., invertebrates have no spinal column; insects have three basic body parts; flowering plants produce flowers and fruits), and use these characteristics to further classify various kinds of plants and animals (*e.g., invertebrates– arthropods – insects; vertebrates – mammals – primates; seed plants – flowering plants – grasses*).

SCIENCE AND TECHNOLOGY - BIODIVERSITY:

1. Relating Science and Technology to Society and the Environment.

1.1 Analyze a local issue related to biodiversity (*e.g., the effects of human activities on urban biodiversity, flooding of traditional Indigenous hunting and gathering areas as a result of dam construction*), taking different points of view into consideration (*e.g., the points of view of members of the local community, business owners, people concerned about the environment, mine owners, local First Nations, Métis, Inuit*), propose action that can be taken to preserve biodiversity, and act on the proposal.

2. Developing Investigation and Communication Skills.

2.3 Use scientific inquiry/research skills to compare the characteristics of organisms within the plant or animal kingdoms (*e.g., compare the characteristics of a fish and a mammal, of coniferous and deciduous trees, of ferns and flowering plants*).

2.5 Use a variety of forms (*e.g., oral, written, graphic, multimedia*) to communicate with different audiences and for a variety of purposes (*e.g., use a graphic organizer to show comparisons between organisms in various communities*).

3.5 Describe interrelationships within species (*e.g., wolves travel in packs to defend their territory, raise their cubs, and hunt large prey*), between species (*e.g., the brightly coloured anemone fish protects its eggs by laying them among the poisonous tentacles of the sea anemone, and in return the fish's bright colours attract prey for the anemone to eat; birds and bees take sustenance from plants and carry pollen between plants*), and between species and their environment (*e.g., algae and water lilies compete for sunlight in a pond*), and explain how these interrelationships sustain biodiversity.

Table 4.1. Curriculum Connections.
Source: Ontario, Ministry of Education, *The Ontario Curriculum: Elementary Grade 6*, 2010.

are no timelines on the lesson plans that have been outlined. It is at the discretion of the teacher to coordinate these activities within a time frame that allows students adequate periods to reflect, create, and conceptualize. However, to illustrate the concept of what a unit plan might look like, we have included a sample plan from the curriculum guide. The premise is that the student has already gone onto the land for Minookum, experienced it, and returned to the classroom. The student and the teacher then work together to reflect on and contextualize the experiences of fishing during Minookum (see Figure 4.6).

By processing our experiences of being on the land, we began to examine how land-based practices might align with the province of Ontario's curriculum. To begin, we reviewed the eight subjects found in the grade six curriculum: Arts, French as a Second Language, Health and Physical Education, Language, Mathematics, Native Languages, Science and Technology, and Social Studies. Following a review of these subject areas, we decided that Health and Physical Education, Science and Technology, Native Languages, Social Studies, Language, and Arts all aligned well with Minookum experiences. It should be noted here that Indigenous Languages curriculum is included in our document because through an immersed and invigorating experience on the land and by learning from Elders and community members who speak Oji-Cree, students will have an integrated experience with their language. However, within the provincial curriculum, the Indigenous Languages program is run based on each school board's discretion. In the curriculum there also is an Indigenous Perspectives document. This document is meant to encourage teachers to include First Nations, Métis, and Inuit content in their classrooms. However, there is a challenge to make the subject meaningful when Indigenous content "is offered in an 'add-on' approach that does not serve the cultural needs of its Indigenous students" (Bell 2011, 392). In contrast, the initiatives put forward by Indigenous communities, such as Wawakapewin, show a desire to move past the "add-on" approach toward a self-determined (Battiste 2011) and culturally relevant curriculum that aligns with provincial or territorial expectations.

Working through each subject, we selected various sections and subsections of the curriculum that were best suited to land-based activities. As demonstrated in Table 4.1, there are two separate columns. Column 1 is allotted to Minookum. The subjects we chose to connect directly to being on the land are listed within column 1. In the second column, we placed curriculum connections that corresponded best with the resources that were developed for the reflection and contextualization of Minookum. It should be emphasized that the numeration that describes each section and subsection of the subjects we chose corresponds directly to Ontario's curriculum documents. Each subject has a different numeration system and also a different way of describing their content.

Conclusion

Historical evidence demonstrates that residential schools and other colonial institutions attempted to disrupt Indigenous subsistence and educational practices by targeting the very foundations of communities and cultures. Even though Indigenous peoples across the country resisted these assimilatory efforts, these strategies had numerous destructive consequences at both individual and community levels. At the heart of these colonial initiatives, there were policies that endorsed the self-proclaimed racial superiority of Euro-Canadians and the colonial government's arrogant assumption that it knew what was best for Indigenous children and communities. As Miller notes, "The problem is that Euro-Canadian society, believing that it knows best or that it couldn't turn control over to Native people, has consistently perverted what Aboriginal people have asked of it in return for sharing the land and its resources of Canada" (1996, 437). In part, these assumptions and their devastating consequences need to be redressed through the integration of land-based curriculum that is led by Indigenous educators for Indigenous children. It is important to stress that our purpose of examining Euro-Canadian and Indigenous pedagogical structures was not to facilitate a process whereby Indigenous methods of knowledge production and transmission could be co-opted into provincial and territorial curriculum streams. Rather, our intention was to understand historically how the two divergent systems have collided, leading to the marginalization of Indigenous knowledge, including land-based subsistence practices. Our central objective was to build a land-based curriculum that privileges Indigenous knowledge and methods and enables Indigenous people to reassert control of their education at regional, local, and community levels.

While we do think that it is possible to meet provincial and territorial curriculum expectations using Indigenous-centred approaches that support local systems of knowledge production as well as cultural and linguistic continuities, questions remain that require further research and analysis. For example, what are the challenges of fully integrating a structure that meets a community's land-based educational needs, but also speaks to the standardized curriculum? How do we implement these curriculum changes at the provincial and territorial levels in ways that respect process, but also ensure that communities are in control of their children's growth and learning? And finally, how can land-based curriculum programs account for and address the gaps in cultural knowledge that were created by colonial education institutions? These are key questions that demand the attention of scholars, policy makers, and education leaders in Indigenous communities.

Our presentation of this land-based curriculum is a starting point for researchers to think critically about how the production and transmission of Indigenous knowledge can be supported by provincial and territorial educational structures. Our suggested model is not an endorsement of a universal approach that can be applied internationally to Indigenous communities or even regionally in Canada. Our model is far too limited in scope to make predictions concerning how easily it can be replicated in different contexts in diverse Indigenous communities. To build a comprehensive land-based curriculum for a particular community and offer productive ways forward, researchers not only need to incorporate Indigenous perspectives, but also to participate in land-based practices. This way they will be able to understand how localized knowledge production and transmission is facilitated by being on the land and by engaging with Elders and other knowledgeable community members. In essence, this chapter calls for researchers to understand these educational needs and the perspectives of leaders and Elders at the most basic level. From our perspective, this can only be accomplished through extensive collaboration, attentive listening to the desires of community members, and active learning and participation in these programs.

Notes

1. As this chapter specifically refers to the isolated region of Northwestern Ontario, it is crucial to acknowledge the residential schools that Indigenous children from these communities would have attended: Cecilia Jeffrey Indian Residential School, Kenora, ON (opened 1900, closed 1966); McIntosh Indian Residential School, Kenora, ON (opened 1924, closed 1969); St. Mary's Indian Residential School, Kenora, ON (opened 1894, closed 1962); Sioux Lookout Indian Residential School and Pelican Lake Day School, Sioux Lookout, ON (opened 1911, closed 1973).

2. For a comprehensive understanding of the Truth and Reconciliation Commission of Canada (TRC) and to read the final reports, including the *Calls to Action*, please see: www.trc.ca.

3. It is critical to acknowledge the community members of Wawakapewin for inviting us into their community to take part in this valuable learning experience. Their commitment to educate their youth using traditional ecological knowledge and land-based practices has in many regards inspired this chapter. *Miigwetch!*

4. It is often the case that in many Indigenous communities across Canada, especially in those with smaller schools, some classrooms include students of several ages. The histories of the negative influences that governmental education institutions have had in some communities have led to low levels of community participation in formalized educational structures. Consequently, it has become a common practice to hold students back from progressing to the next grade due to low records of attendance and sometimes a lack of academic achievement based on minimum provincial or territorial standards. The end result is classrooms with an age span that on average is wider than in many communities throughout the country.

5. Gruenewald (2003) connects critical pedagogy of place to curriculum arguing that it increases student engagement through multidisciplinary, experiential, and intergenerational learning.

6. The Canadian Council on Learning report on the state of Aboriginal learning in Canada notes that "learning is the purpose of the life journey that begins at birth and continues throughout one's lifetime" (2009, 6). This concept, that life is learning, challenges the structured formal setting of education.

References

Alfred, Gerald R. 1995. *Heeding the Voices of Our Ancestors: Kahnawake Mohawk Politics and the Rise of Native Nationalism*. Toronto: Oxford University Press.

Anderson, Leighton. 2011. Personal interview. 27 May.

Anuik, Jonathan, Marie Battiste, and Priscilla George. 2010. "Learning from Promising Programs and Applications in Nourishing the

Learning Spirit." *Canadian Journal of Native Education* 33 (1): 63–82.

Barman, Jean, Yvonne Hébert, and Don McCaskill, eds. 1986. *Indian Education in Canada, Volume 1: The Legacy.* Vancouver: University of British Columbia Press.

———. 1987. *Indian Education in Canada, Volume 2: The Challenge.* Vancouver: University of British Columbia Press.

Battiste, Marie. 2002. *Indigenous Knowledge and Pedagogy in First Nation Education: A Literature Review with Recommendations.* Prepared for the National Working Group on Education and the Minister of Indian Affairs, Indian and Northern Affairs Canada. Ottawa: Apamuwek Institute.

———. 2011. "Curriculum Reform through Constitutional Reconciliation of Indigenous Knowledge." In *Contemporary Studies in Canadian Curriculum: Principles, Portraits, and Practices,* edited by Darren Stanley and Kelly Young, 287–312. Calgary, AB: Detselig Enterprises.

Bell, Nicole. 2011. "Creating Shared Understandings: Meeting Indigenous Education Needs." In *Contemporary Studies in Canadian Curriculum: Principles, Portraits, and Practices,* edited by Darren Stanley and Kelly Young, 375–98. Calgary, AB: Detselig Enterprises.

Bracken, Christopher. 1997. *The Potlatch Papers: A Colonial Case Study.* Chicago: University of Chicago Press.

Cajete, Gregory. 1994. *Look to the Mountain: An Ecology of Indigenous Education.* Skyland, NC: Kívakí Press.

Canadian Council on Learning. 2009. *The State of Aboriginal Learning in Canada: A Holistic Approach to Measuring Success.* Ottawa: Canadian Council on Learning.

Cruikshank, Julie. 2005. *Do Glaciers Listen? Local Knowledge, Colonial Encounters, and Social Imagination.*

Vancouver: University of British Columbia Press.

Curwen Doige, Linda A. 2003. "A Missing Link: Between Traditional Aboriginal Education and the Western System of Education." *Canadian Journal of Native Education* 27 (2): 144–60.

Frogg, Simon. 2011. Personal interview. 25 May.

Gruenewald, David A. 2003. "The Best of Both Worlds: A Critical Pedagogy of Place." *Educational Researcher* 32 (4): 3–12.

Haig-Brown, Celia. 1988. *Resistance and Renewal: Surviving the Indian Residential School.* Vancouver: Tillacum Library.

Hickling-Hudson, Anne, and Roberta Ahlquist. 2003. "Contesting the Curriculum in the Schooling of Indigenous Children in Australia and the United States: From Eurocentrism to Culturally Powerful Pedagogies." *Comparative Education Review* 47 (1): 64–89.

Kana'iaupuni, Shawn Malia. 2005. "Ka'akalai ku kanaka: A Call for Strengths-Based Approaches from a Native Hawaiian Perspective." *Educational Researcher* 34 (5): 32–38.

Kovach, Margaret. 2009. *Indigenous Methodologies: Characteristics, Conversations, and Contexts.* Toronto: University of Toronto Press.

Kovacs, Patricia. 2009. *Synthesis Report of the Aboriginal Learning Knowledge Centre's Literature Reviews: Responsive Educational Systems.* Saskatoon, SK: Canadian Council on Learning and Aboriginal Learning Knowledge Centre.

Mason, Courtney W. 2012. "Consuming the Physical and Cultural Practices of Aboriginal Peoples: Spaces of Exchange, Conflict and (Post)colonial Power Relations." In *The Role of Sports in the Formation of Personal Identities: Studies in Community Loyalties,* edited by John E. Hughson, Clive

Palmer, and Fiona Skillen, 167–90. London: Edwin Mellen Press.

———. 2014. *Spirits of the Rockies: Reasserting An Indigenous Presence in Banff National Park.* Toronto: University of Toronto Press.

Meekis, Archie. 2011. Personal interview. 28 May.

Meyer, Planulani Aluli. 2008. "Indigenous and Authentic: Hawaiian Epistemology and the Triangulation of Meaning." In *Handbook of Critical and Indigenous Methodologies,* edited by Norman K. Denzin, Yvonna S. Lincoln, and Linda Tuhiwai Smith, 217–32. Los Angeles: SAGE Publishers.

Miller, J.R. 1996. *Shingwauk's Vision: A History of Native Residential Schools.* Toronto: University of Toronto Press.

Milloy, John S. 1999. *A National Crime: The Canadian Government and the Residential School System, 1879–1986.* Winnipeg: University of Manitoba Press.

Mosby, Ian. 2013. "Administering Colonial Science: Nutrition Research and Human Biomedical Experimentation in Aboriginal Communities and Residential Schools, 1942–1952." *Histoire Sociale/ Social History* 46 (91): 145–72.

Nanokeesic, Jeremiah. 2011. Personal interview, interpreted by S. Frogg. 26 May.

Ohmagari, Kayo, and Fikret Berkes. 1997. "Transmission of Indigenous Knowledge and Bush Skills among the Western James Bay Cree Women of Sub-Arctic Canada." *Human Ecology* 25 (2): 197–222.

Ontario. Ministry of Education. 2010. *The Ontario Curriculum: Elementary Grade 6.*

Pearce, Tristan, Harold Wright, Roland Notaina, Adam Kudlak, Barry Smit, James D. Ford, and Christopher Furgal. 2011. "Transmission of Indigenous Knowledge and Land Skills among Inuit Men in Ulukhaktok, Northwest Territories, Canada." *Human Ecology* 39 (3): 271–88.

Redwing Saunders, Sabrina E., and Susan M. Hill. 2007. "Native Education and In-Classroom Coalition-Building: Factors and Models in Delivering an Equitous Authentic Education." *Canadian Journal of Education* 30 (4): 1015–45.

Smith, Graham H. 2009. "Mai i te Maramatanga, ki te Putanga Mai o te Tahuritanga: From Conscientization to Transformation." In *Social Justice, Peace and Environmental Education: Transformative Standard,* edited by Julie Andrzejewski, Marta Baltodano, and Linda Symcox, 19–28. London: Routledge.

Smith, Linda Tuhiwai. 1999. *Decolonizing Methodologies: Research and Indigenous Peoples.* London: Zed Books.

Snow, John. 2005. *These Mountains are Our Sacred Places: The Story of the Stoney People.* Calgary: Fifth House Publishing.

Stiffarm, Lenore A. 1998. *As We See–: Aboriginal Pedagogy.* Saskatoon: University Extension Press.

Swan, I. 1998. "Modelling: An Aboriginal Approach." In *As We See–: Aboriginal Pedagogy,* edited by Lenore A. Stiffarm, 77–85. Saskatoon: University Extension Press.

Takano, Takako. 2005. "Connections with the Land: Land-Skills Courses in Igloolik, Nunavut." *Ethnography* 6 (4): 463–86.

Chapter Five

PIMATISIWIN

*Women, Wellness, and Land-Based
Practices for Omushkego Youth*

Today, Indigenous communities are familiar with the challenges of equi-
table food access, sustainable land-based practices, health, cost of living,
structural discrimination, youth suicide, and loss of cultural knowledge.
As revealed in Chapter 4, intergenerational stressors, including residential schools and displacements from ancestral lands, have undermined
individual and community well-being. Still, Indigenous peoples' connection to the land has long played a vital role in sustaining their kinship
structures, cultural practices, and subsistence economies. Therefore, it is
this connection that provides the impetus to revitalize land-based practices—in this instance *Pimatisiwin*, the Cree holistic conception of life.
This chapter presents knowledge gathered in a research project with the
Moose Cree First Nation,[1] in Moose Factory, Ontario, which is located on
an island at the southern tip of James Bay. The people of this community
are known as the Omushkegowuk. This chapter demonstrates the ways
in which Omushkego efforts to restore peoples' connections to the land
have helped the community to respond to colonial conditions and to promote cultural continuance. I begin with an examination of a land-based
initiative for youth and discuss the role Omushkego women play in restoring cultural practices. The chapter then explores how reconnecting to the
land restores wholeness, fosters cultural continuance, recognizes women's
contributions to community well-being, and increases food security. The

results I present in this chapter strengthen the importance of investing in land-based initiatives.

Project Context

It is important to begin by outlining the nature of my involvement with the Moose Cree community as this project unfolded. Moose Cree was one of the first communities engaged in a pilot project, Right to Play Canada (RTP), delivering recreational programming for young Indigenous people. In November 2011, I participated in an RTP hockey-for-development camp as part of a research partnership with the University of Ottawa's School of Human Kinetics. My role was to evaluate the development of RTP programming for Indigenous youth. At one of the many RTP training sessions, held at a Tim Horton Children's Foundation camp, the Moose Cree mentor at the time, Darryl Dick, expressed interest in collaborating on a unique research project, either as part of RTP's programming or alongside it. In that initial exchange, he gave me a video called *Project George: Reconnecting Youth to the Land.* Our exchanges led to an invitation for me to attend the August 2013 Moose Cree First Nation Gathering of Our People (GOOP), to learn more about Moose Cree culture. I spent two weeks in the community, assisting the John R. Delaney Youth Centre staff in their youth leadership program. Although there were differing views of the structure and governance of RTP within the community, emphasis on reconnecting youth to the land emerged as a common theme. Many people, including the youth, expressed the need to learn the ways of the land, to be on the land, and to make this connection to the land relevant within youth-centred initiatives. It quickly became evident that the land was at the heart of the people and furthermore at the heart of *Pimatisiwin.* These conversations with the Omushkegowuk redirected my initial research question to a broader vision that could support the youth's connection to the land and advocate for the community's engagement in land-based activities.

As a result of these formal and informal exchanges, a project called *Pimatisiwin: Healthy Living for Youth* was conceived. It encouraged youth and Elder participation in existing land-based initiatives, such as Project George, and highlighted the importance of land-based skills and *Pimatisiwin* teachings. My role was to learn about the land-based activities—how they were organized by the community and what were the various desired outcomes of participating in them. To carry out my research, I spent two months in the community. I assisted with youth centre planning, participated in and volunteered at community events and locally led conferences, took excursions with families, and attended cultural ceremonies such as sweat lodges. I participated in a three-day on-the-land excursion with fifteen young people, three female Elders, two educators, and the camp owner. I worked out of the community's youth centre, which helped me to build relationships with members of the Moose Cree community. Relationship building through community participation is a feature of my own Métis and Cree kinship system. As a Métis scholar participating in community-based research, I believe it is paramount to be grounded in my own history and, in part, to bear responsibility for the interests, dreams, struggles, and aspirations of the Métis and Cree people. My research included participatory observation, visits, and forty unstructured and semi-structured conversations with the staff of Project George, the camp owner, the chief and members of the Moose Cree Band Council, youth centre workers, Elders, health care professionals, youth leaders, and educators. A reciprocal participation in each other's lives led to meaningful conversations and to ongoing, community-based projects. This type of research philosophy is transformative, exploratory, and lived: it invites openness, trust, and flexibility.

The Omushkego People: The People of the Land

For millennia, the Omushkego lifestyle involved seasonal movement, adapted to hunting and harvesting. The people lived a semi-nomadic existence, making best use of the abundant land and water, food, and material resources. As depicted throughout this book with other Indigenous peoples across Canada, the Omushkego of the Moose Cree First Nation were forced to modify their land-based culture as a result of colonial disruptions. The development of the fur trade depleted food and other resources, forcing people in the region to become dependent on Western technologies, food, and material goods. Compounding this dependency were the forced introductions of reserves and residential schools, impositions that transformed a way of life intimately tied to the land.

In the twenty-first century the Moose Cree live with this legacy of dependency. Even so, they are fighting to reclaim land-based cultural practices and to incorporate them into contemporary life. This resurgence has led the community members to proudly share their knowledge of cultural practices—in particular, practices centred on food, language, rituals, and gatherings. The associate executive director of the Moose Cree First Nation, Bertha Sutherland, explains that the land "urges each person to remember and to reclaim who they are" (Sutherland 2014, Personal interview).[2] She and many other community members refer to regaining their inherent rights, culture, and lifestyles as part of the process of reconnecting to the land.

The Moose Cree often describe their connection to the land as bonding them to their ancestors, who lived and relied on the land. The Cree way of life is typically characterized by land-based activities, such as hunting, gathering, trapping, and fishing, but it also includes other aspects. Lawrence Martin, Omuskego grand chief, elaborates on the Cree relationship to the land: "It refers to the idea that we are extensions of the land, our lives are directly linked to it, for water, food, and dreams" (Martin 2015). When describing land-based activities, community members often talked about feeling a profound connection to their surroundings. Allen Sailors, director of Health Services, explained that the connection to the land needed to be experienced and, more importantly, felt. He observed that this feeling can be strengthened by time spent on the land and spoke of the land's power of healing: "The land and that connection changes you. . . . The land is not to try to possess or to rip apart, it is a living creature, and your whole attitude changes. That's why whatever you take from the land, you got to put something back. When you have that connection, you learn how to respect the land, and you realize there is that healing power that comes from the land" (Sailors 2014). Nathan Cheechoo, a young man and father, shared his feelings toward the land, "I believe in the power of the land, because I felt it, time and time again" (N. Cheechoo 2013). For Nathan and other community members engaged in land-based activities, the land is about learning discipline, commitment, dedication, and determination to live. In this context, the physical and mental effort of finding a moose, looking for tracks, using one's voice as a means to call the geese, preparing the camp, staying warm, melting snow, setting up a hunting blind, and getting up early are the necessary everyday tasks required to feed one's family.

Others explained to me how the land once was, and is now again, the natural forum to teach history—what the ancestors did and how they survived through harvesting, hunting, fishing, and gathering. Kiersten Wapachee, a young woman working as a youth leader, stated that her grandmother seeks to instill what she calls a "traditional feeling" in her grandchildren. This is to ensure that they do not lose their way within the mainstream educational systems. She explained that her grandmother talks about the past and her father talks about the present. Kiersten's grandmother also taught her how to pluck geese, cook bannock, and survive in the bush. The young woman further expressed her fear of what would happen if Elders did not teach traditional knowledge to the youth: "If they stop teaching us what it was like back then, then it will be a different world" (Wapachee 2013). Clearly, some members are worried regarding the lack of knowledge about the land and the disconnection of generations in the community. Drug and alcohol use among youth, both indicators of alienation, is also a common concern. Earl Cheechoo, deputy chief, offered another significant contribution to this conversation: "Youth are in a spiritual crisis. They don't know how, or who, to pray to. We think that we need to change, but no, we are okay. We make it so hard for ourselves, and we are hard on ourselves. We are decolonizing our thinking. We have our own laws. We are challenging our government policies. We are returning to customary laws" (2014). Community members are responding to these concerns by making a greater effort to reconnect youth with the land through land-based activities that engage young people and foster interactive, experiential learning. Paul Linklater, vice principal of Delores D. Echum Composite School, explains: "The youth have to go on the land and interact with it. This is the key to youth participation. That is how rich we are in our culture. . . . We engage and interact and have the knowledge of the land. We have to go back to our roots. Our youth need more direction" (2014). These deliberate efforts to reintegrate land-based practices in families, schools, and through wider community initiatives have important implications for what Karen Pine Cheechoo, a grandmother, explains is the lack of understanding of what it means to be *illewuk*, or a Cree person. She says, "Without the connection to language and the land, one loses touch with where they came from, and how they lived" (K. P. Cheechoo 2014).

Concerns specific to youth well-being have led to the development of a Youth Services Department. The department's objectives are to improve youth networking in the Mushkegowuk Region and to increase youth engagement, youth leadership, knowledge, and skills. The grand chief of the region explained that to achieve sustainable youth well-being, Cree youth teachings need to be revitalized. He referred me to a recent report, posted on the Mushkegowuk Council website, containing the results of a community-based inquiry into suicides. The community's approach—in this case to an intergenerational legacy of colonization leading to youth suicides and addictions—is a grassroots response. Project George is an example of such a land-based initiative emerging from a need to help the youth reconnect to the land.

Project George: Reconnecting Youth to the Land

Project George is a land-based initiative that began in 2009. Charlie Cheechoo, now Project George coordinator, remembered listening to the Elder George E. Eechum, who was concerned that the youth lacked physical activities to divert them from video games, drugs, and alcohol. A few years later, an eighteen-year-old young man, also named George, approached Charlie and asked him to take him fishing. After their fishing trip, the young man asked if Charlie would take out more youth, if he had the equipment to do so. Stan Louttit, former Grand Chief, explained that many young people in the community wanted to participate in these types of activities but were unable, due to the expense and other circumstances beyond their control. Charlie was able to acquire the gear and three months later he took a group of six youth to his friend's camp. This was how Project George started. In 2009, the community experienced a youth suicide crisis, making it even more apparent that youth were facing considerable challenges and that something needed to be done to help them. The positive feedback to youth participation in the land-based activities Charlie was offering boosted support for formalizing what became known as Project George.

The mission statement of Project George is to bring at-risk youth into the bush, and to help them connect with the land and with Cree traditions, for the purposes of recovery and personal growth. The project's objective is to improve the lives of youth who have been affected by the trauma of poverty, family breakdown, and suicide. The initiative facilitates the learning of Cree skills such as fishing, trapping, hunting, and setting up camp, and values such as caring for the camp and for each other through experiential and intergenerational learning on the land. In its first years of operation, Project George was funded by donations from local organizations and corporations. These contributions covered the expenses of camping equipment, food, lodge rental, travel costs, equipment repair, and salaries. Moose Cree First Nation has also subsidized Project George, by covering the salary of the program coordinator and providing an office space and computer in the John Delaney Youth Centre. Since 2009, Project George has been able to bring 200 young people camping for three to ten days at a time. From 2011 to 2013, grants from Ontario First Nations Limited Partnership enabled an increase of youth participation in land-based activities. Other collaborations with band members, such as William Tozer, have provided more camp space for Project George to facilitate its land-based excursions.

Project George serves the community's youth, both male and female. In some instances, entire families participate, revitalizing cultural knowledge connected with the harvesting of traditional foods. There is an element of spontaneity to Project George trips. As Charlie explained, "there is no formal kind of structure, and even when you're out there, there is no formal structure" (C. Cheechoo 2014). Unlike the more ordered and often rigid programming typical in the South, Project George is relaxed and fluid. As a result, William has noticed the difference in young people's behaviours on the second day of being at the camp: "A natural bonding occurs just letting youth visit, share and be together. Their days are not filled with keeping them active and entertained. We like to keep it simple. . . . We are here to learn the land and from the land" (Tozer 2014). Charlie explains that they are guided by the land, as well as by the youth:

> The weather dictates what we do, so it looks different every
> time. The kids look forward to it . . . most of the time it is
> them that decide what to do. Let's go fishing . . . ok let's go.
> What are we doing in the morning? I don't know: it depends
> on the weather . . . let's eat breakfast first. One of things I

really fight against is structure. When we take our own ideas in the bush, you don't plan activities, you just do them. You have an idea of what you are going to do. That's what I take to the project. First of all it depends on the weather . . . we're not going to leave if it's forty below. (C. Cheechoo 2014)

Although the project may appear unstructured, some structure unequivocally exists. And there is an element of surrender to the land, rather than control over it.

Those working for Project George have a responsibility to give back to the community, for example by bringing firewood to the Elders and assisting in communal events. The program teaches youth the importance of giving back by sharing their catch with their families, the community, and the Elders who are not able to go on the land. These actions speak to a way of life that does not merely bolster self-confidence and self-esteem, but also teaches the responsibility of being helpers and role models who instill dignity. The project environment accommodates young men and women, ensuring meaningful, safe, and successful learning. Safety was often mentioned in conversation, as it became a concern, given environmental changes and the increase in youth participation. In addition, training in first aid, chainsaw and firearms safety, driving on snow and ice, and Moose Cree versions of safety and survival courses were offered through Project George.

Project leaders and youth workers believe that land-based initiatives have reduced young people's consumption of alcohol and drugs. Having gained knowledge of surviving on the land, the Project George youth workers now also feel that they are part of something bigger than themselves. Donovan Cheechoo, who has been working with Project George for three years, openly shared how he felt on the land: "I feel like the ancestors are there with you and watching. I belong to them, and they to me" (D. Cheechoo 2014). During the project, youth workers set up the hunting blinds and help build the cabins, tent frames, and lean-tos. They show the younger participants survival skills, such as tracking and setting rabbit snares, catching and cleaning fish, and hunting and field-dressing moose. The youth workers feel that this knowledge has helped the younger men and women to know and benefit from their traditions and culture.

Although Project George began small, it has been successful in providing youth the opportunity to experience, to heal, and to learn about life in the bush. With a long-term vision in mind, strategic and financial plans were developed in 2013 to establish Project George as a permanent outdoor community education program. The youth workers equally shared their idea of this initiative as well as their hopes that land-based programming will continue and that more youth and Elders will take part. They want to help other Indigenous communities create similar programs for youth who are unable to participate in land-based activities. They spoke of the importance of updating and maintaining the Project George Facebook page, and of offering consistent, seasonal land-based programming. Donovan shared his experience of a three-day paddling trip up the Moose River, where he and others learned from two professionals how to camp, and how to paddle and ride the rapids. He dreams of more trips of a similar nature. The community engaged the youth in assessing the value of land-based initiatives. Some of the evaluation questions that emerged in our conversation were: "What did it feel like? How was your experience? What did you learn? Would you go again?" The helpers further hoped that Project George would own its hunting camp and create its own logo, based on the theme of reconnecting with the land.

In Moose Cree First Nation, the young people's engagement in land-based practices instigates an array of emotions and enthusiasm. Such engagement addresses the community's concerns related to youth well-being and sustainable programming. Recognizing that social challenges are not isolated to youth, Project George has grown to include the community. Despite the fact that men coordinate and run the program, women play an integral role in its development. The next section will highlight women's contributions to Project George and their views on the importance of land-based programming.

Women's Contribution to Land-Based Initiatives

As the project evolved, female Elders and other women in the community became involved because of their unique knowledge and prudent management of the household. Their land-based expertise became essential to effectively manage certain aspects of the program. The involvement of women led to the enrichment of land-based initiatives in ways that welcomed young women. Their participation promoted collaboration with several organizations in the community, including the local churches, the John Delaney Youth Centre, and Moose Factory's schools. Women also provided different methods of learning, teaching, and meaning related to the land. In Cree, *eskoe* means women and is described in the context of female-male relationships, principles, roles, and responsibilities. Lawrence Martin explains how they go together: "[*Eskoe*] is further an abbreviation to other words that relate to life, to time, and to fire. In terms of *eskoe*'s connection to life, it is one who stays with life for its entirety. In terms of time, it refers to responsibility. In terms of fire, it has to do with giving life and taking life. When describing female, it has nothing to do with woman, rather it is the one who shows care and who nurtures" (2014). He went on to say that *eskoe* could be a child, a moose, or a plant. Given the larger goal of re-establishing youth's connection to the land, many of the Cree values are tied to the balancing of the male-female principles. In the context of Project George, the women not only made this community initiative more culturally relevant, but they further enriched the experience by increasing its accessibility and knowledge base. Their stories of the land are unique to their experiences as Omushkego women. Their concern with a broader meaning of land is different from men's. Both perspectives are needed to ensure the well-being of the whole community.

Over the course of a particular land-based excursion, I observed how the women provided care, food, instruction, and traditional knowledge to the youth and to their helpers. As they instructed, the women never once raised their voices, blew whistles, gave orders, or established rules or punitive consequences, nor did they need to. Their presence and commitment to the young people felt grounding and reassuring. They directed the kitchen and took care of all the meals and the warmth of the lodge, which was our living space. As they prepared the food, they shared stories and laughter. One Elder, Agnes Wesley-Corston, taught the youth and educators how to skin a rabbit. They all huddled around the kitchen table and listened attentively. I took photos and recorded this very important lesson. As she skinned the rabbit, she told anecdotes of her life and conveyed the ways in which almost all parts of animals were consumed. She explained that even the rabbit ears were put on the fire and eaten as treats, she laughed, and drew a parallel with potato chips. She also discussed the non-food-related value of all parts of the animal, for instance rabbit fur, which was used to make coats and was also put inside socks or gloves for warmth.

In conversation about issues related to the land, the women spoke about their concerns with the contamination of food today and how this affects the physical life and the minds of young people. They spoke of life in the bush, and how their mothers taught them to clean geese. Similar to the discussion in Chapter 3 around the extensive hunting or harvesting by Indigenous communities, women emphasized how it was necessary to make use of all parts. Elder Mary Cheechoo-Linklater said, "We even clean the heads and wings, and we used the feathers to make comforters. We used all parts. We used to clean all the guts too and make goose lard. We had a good, hard life. The only thing we threw out was the poop . . . almost everything was saved" (Cheechoo-Linklater 2014). The women also spoke about the medicines of the land—for example, how their grandmothers would get sap from different trees to heal illnesses. Two women in their seventies remembered clearly the journey from Moose Factory to their families' traditional territories in the bush. They talked about how simple their life was in the bush and how they relied on the land for most of their subsistence.

These women worried about what the youth were facing today in the community. They felt that young people would need to learn to live on the land again because of the problems with food contamination and with the way the world was changing. Agnes commented, "That's why it is good to bring the children out; they get to taste the food we used to eat" (Wesley-Corston 2014). By eating food from the land, young people establish a relationship with their surroundings and become grounded in the knowledge of a particular place. Traditional food-related practices evoke a sense of belonging, often relayed through stories. The women provided additional knowledge about relating to the environment in a way that ensured an empathetic connection to the past, present, and the future.

Land-based food practices are collective experiences where all community members can participate in their unique capacity. I observed this collective aspect when Agnes kindly instructed her son to offer two geese to the camp excursion. The geese were prepared and cooked over an open fire in a teepee. All the while, the women shared stories. Learning was ongoing, and the women restored a connection to the land by embodying the knowledge and the generous spirit of the land. The benefits of connecting to the land extended beyond the youth, to Elders and the community. The women repeatedly shared their enthusiasm for being a part of the land-based excursions. Mary said, "it helps us to remember our life" (Cheechoo-Linklater 2014). The simple act of eating berries from the land evoked the memory of learning from their own mothers and grandmothers. It also brought back memories of what was lost through residential schools. In 1855, Horden Hall Residential School was established in Moose Factory, mainly enrolling students from the traditional Omushkego territories. Some of these women's relatives attended the school, and as a result they did not learn the ways of the land. As was acknowledged in Chapter 4, for many people in the community, the residential school severed their connection to the land. As mothers, aunties, sisters, and grandmothers, these women now help youth to get to know the Cree values and ways of life. They are confident that by simply "being out on the land that traditional knowledge would stick to their insides because the land is part of them too" (Cheechoo-Linklater 2014).

For quite some time I have reflected on the words of Karen Pine Cheechoo. One evening, over tea, she shared with me her journey as a young woman reconnecting with the land during the 1970s. She referred to this time as waking up the Elders. Ironically, she recounted that "the Elders were not sleeping; they simply needed a space to educate us" (K. P. Cheechoo 2014). The land was historically the context for learning and teaching. She further emphasized that it was not necessarily *what* Elders taught, but *how* they taught:

> There was a lot of language saying we have to wake up our
> Elders. . . . So we went and they started educating us [out of
> the community, on the land]. All of us women, we would sit
> together and have to clean 100 geese. We'd sit and clean all
> day. The next day, we'd be cooking all day. We'd do different
> foods and feed the guests we had invited. These men would
> sit and tell stories. They'd show young people how to make
> a net. It became a community of learning. It was like the

spirit of our community began to grow. There we felt the community spirit. . . . They would talk to us about our relationship and it would be done in humour. Women's work and men's work doing their thing. There was always lots of communication. It wasn't so much what they said, it was a lot of how they said. It wasn't the words, but it was how they said it. How they said it made more sense, it made people feel invited into that conversation. (K. P. Cheechoo 2014)

When reflecting on women's unique contribution to the community, there is a tendency to focus on what they do and what they teach, as opposed to the ways in which women do it. I mention this as it appears to be vital in conversations about the importance of land-based learning and the involvement of Elders. The transference of knowledge goes beyond learning specific skills. It is about belonging to a people and a place, having a respectful relationship with the land, and knowing that the path of self-reliance requires a connection to food, animals, and cultural values. These women lived and embodied what Sailors explained as the Cree concept of the four human laws taught by the land itself—kindness, strength, sharing, and honesty (Sailors 2014).

Impacts of Reconnecting to the Land
The voices of the people prompt a deeper consideration of the consequences of reconnecting to the land. In this section, I will explore these consequences. A priority in my research was to determine what was important to the community in relation to their experience and knowledge of reconnecting to the land. Four main impacts, invariably woven together, emerged in the community conversations: (1) restoration of a sense of wholeness through kinship systems, (2) fostering of cultural continuance through stories, (3) recognition of women's contribution to community well-being, and (4) increased food security. By no means are these four concerns exhaustive. They do however offer an indication of the possible impacts of reconnecting to the land.

Connecting individuals to land-based practices and values restores the Cree sense of wholeness, by reinforcing kinship systems comprising human and non-human animals, plants, stories, dreams, and rituals.

The communal ways of being on, and with, the land also yield a collective strength that displaces individualism and social isolation. As I witnessed through Project George, there is no overarching authoritative body governing land-based practices. While leadership and facilitation exist, collective engagement sets up and maintains the camp. Community members strongly believe that being on the land enhances the feeling and knowledge that you are part of the land. Although it is necessary in a contemporary context to inform young people of the logic behind their activities, there is a general feeling that there exists an inner knowing, which will be stimulated on the land. The land heightens the senses, as well as intuition. Consequently, reconnecting to the land is about survival, preserving a sacred way of life, and restoring a sense of belonging.

This spirit of belonging does not only exist in the bush or on the land. It extends itself to enhance one's engagement in, and reflection on, community life. According to Allen Sailors, "It is about being together. It changes how we understand each other. When you are out on the land, you think about how you live in community, how you act and how you interact. You start to think about that when you are out there" (Sailors 2014). Repeatedly people asserted that the land provides individuals with the essential elements from which to draw strength in daily life. While the ways of connecting to land differ in the community, feeling at home on the land was an often-repeated conversational theme. All generations stated that a feeling of peace, grounding, and stillness brought a welcomed pause to modern-day demands and responsibilities. Asynee Apay Shko, a Cree mother and health care professional, explained that for her the land is a place to reconnect with herself. "That's what I do when I get back from the city . . . I feel called to go to the land because I feel displaced. . . . I need to go ground myself. I talk and sing to the trees. . . . I know they like the songs. It draws positive stuff around me. My children are taught why that is where they need to go" (Shko 2014).

In conversations, community members expressed a deep desire to live in harmony with the land, in the ways of their ancestors. Coming to know oneself through the knowledge of ancestors—how they lived and where they came from—was important to the community. The generations of people who were taught by their grandparents, and who remain engaged in land-based initiatives, have become crucial mentors. As part of the land-based activities, the Elders shared history and their knowledge of what it meant to live on the land. The knowledge of where to find food and medicine played a role in sustaining self-reliant and active lifestyles. As Elder Agnes Wesley-Corston explained, they would never sit idle on the land: "You had to get your food and even your medication. You would make poultice from the land. My grandfather would get some sap from different trees. I had impetigo for a month, my mom got poplar tree buds, cooked them on the stove, and it went away in three days" (2014). The Elders' stories were often motivational. Going back to the land evoked for many people the desire to reconnect with their physical life, setting up camp and gathering wood, water, and medicines. In addition, knowing one's identity in relation to land, and to one's relatives, inspired young people to want to know more—of their history, language, teachings, and stories.

Storytelling is a common Cree method of learning and teaching about survival. There is strength in those old stories. The stories are told over and over again. In conversations, time and again, Elders emphasized that being on the land provides an uninterrupted time and space to communicate knowledge and teachings through stories. Many community members provided examples of the types of stories shared, for instance, as they sat in the blind during the spring goose-hunting season. The stories explained people's connection to the geese, hunting strategies, the geese's flying patterns, and how the geese offer their lives for the nourishment of the people. Many community members stressed that, in addition to teaching and learning, stories facilitate intergenerational bonds between relatives. In this context, Sailors further suggested that the land shaped the conversations that emerged: "You start talking, and that is the healing, when we talk. And sometimes a child may want to know the history of their family, who was their grandparents, what did they do, how did they survive. . . . You pass on survival skills to the youth. So if they ever get stuck when they are alone, they will know what to do. They don't have to be afraid of anything out there" (2014). Through stories and legends, family members taught one another again about being self-sufficient, aware of survival strategies, and sensitive to the diverse challenges that may arise.

The stories of the Omushkego people inevitably carry the pain and tensions of lived experiences. These too are increasingly being shared in culturally safe contexts or in the privacy of home. As people learn through their kinship system, Indigenous knowledge disrupts Western-based systems that focus on and promote individual success and the nuclear family. Stories shift the relational dynamics within families and, more broadly, within the life of the community.

Reconnecting to the land does more than increase food access or engage community members in a process. It awakens cultural practices and knowledge expressed and embodied in the land, language, and stories. This knowledge can often be shared very naturally when plucking geese, skinning rabbits, sitting in blinds, gathering and preparing medicines, and setting up fishing nets. Stories hold timeless forms of instruction on how to live in accordance with Cree ways of life. For instance, stories of the land teach that well-being is not an individual goal, but rather a collective responsibility. One story shared by Arlene Faries, a mother and storyteller, further demonstrates one of the ways kinship systems restore a sense of wholeness and cultural continuance, the latter being inextricably linked to stories of the land. The story she shared involves a young boy who has run away to the forest because he felt he was not good enough. Eventually, he gets lost in the forest. Faries explains how a large grey songbird, Whiskeyjack, well-known as the reporter of the forest, sees the lost boy. Whiskeyjack remembers that they had forgotten to give the boy his spirit name and reports this information to all its forest relatives. They sing the boy a song embodying his spirit name. They then tell him to go home, reassuring him that he will be a good hunter. It is believed that there is strength in the spirit name, as it guides one's actions. In the story, through his interaction with the forest and its animals, the boy gains purpose and finds his place in the community.

Reconnecting to the land has also helped Moose Cree people better understand their roles and responsibilities in affirming the ancient values and principles of *Pimatisiwin*—the life journey in relation to cycles of life and nature. This knowledge is being revitalized in the community to sustain the healing and well-being of families. Christina Linklater, a mother and a health care professional, participated in the Cree traditional walking-out ceremony. This specific rite of passage relates to children's first steps and their connection to the land, the animals, the water, and the life that will sustain them. For an entire year, the child is kept off the land. After a year, the family and community gather to witness, to feast, and to celebrate the child's first steps on the land. Linklater explained what the ceremony meant to her:

> It gave me a sense of purpose knowing where I came from.
> . . . To know that I would have the strength to get where I
> am going someday. I know it's part of my role to do these
> ceremonies, and it is my role to ensure that my children will
> know what was shared with me. It was a promise to keep
> that alive for them. And that life is precious . . . that they
> will journey and it will be hard sometimes, but there will
> always be a support system for them, and you can always go
> to the land for healing, . . . for prayer, and for meditation. (C.
> Linklater 2014)

Rites of passage such as placenta burials and walking out, snowshoe, and moontime ceremonies were almost lost as a result of residential schools. Their revival has been made possible because some families secretly maintained these practices in intimate family settings. The ceremonies are only now making their way back into the community.

How women transmit and contribute to the continuity of Cree ways of life is evident in land-based practices. Also, through reconnecting to the land, women are now reclaiming their prominent role in sustaining family and community well-being. There is a harrowing concern that, as a result of residential schools, Elders have forgotten how and what to communicate in order to preserve cultural continuity. Land-based practices were once related to teaching and learning Cree parenting. Despite the disruption of intergenerational transmission of parenting skills, grandmothers remain role models. In my conversations with people about their connection with the land, community members expressed that they thought of their grandmothers and often prayed to them during difficult times. Given the lack of resources and unavailability of female Elders, to provide apprenticeship (which is life-long), a circle of Omushkego women are helping each other to restore their families' and their grandmothers' ways. Asynee Apay Shko explains that through ceremony, ancient teachings, and prayer, they are connecting the circle of knowledge and, in her words, "bringing things together and being role models for others" (2014). Being on the land and participating in land-based practices is helping them to learn how to care for themselves again and how to care for their families differently. Awareness that the community will not heal until women and their families heal is emerging in the community's consciousness. As a result, some of the women have identified a need to develop land-based initiatives specific to young women. Their respective connections to the land have helped them recognize their spiritual and creative force in sustaining these critical links.

This awareness has motivated women to become active in their communities. Women are reclaiming their rightful place, gathering knowledge and teachings. They are taking greater leadership roles as grandmothers, mothers, aunties, and sisters. Their efforts, as Earl Cheechoo shares, are not going unnoticed: "Women are going to take the leading role in our healing journey. I see within the community they are really standing out. You know they are talking. Their voices are getting stronger. All these strong women, which is why we are who we are today" (2014). Western systems of thinking rendered Indigenous women powerless, ignored their voices, knowledge, and important role in ensuring community well-being (Anderson 2011). But land-based initiatives and the teachings of *Pimatisiwin* have awakened their physical, emotional, social, and spiritual connection to land, identity, and relationships.

From a practical perspective, land-based initiatives have also resulted in increased food security in the Moose Cree First Nation. Local food procurement, through youth-centre initiatives like Project George, has offered community members opportunities to improve land-based skills and regain confidence in their ability to provide for themselves. In other words, the capacity to feed and to nourish their families has strengthened the Omushkego people's sense of autonomy and further restored a sense of trust in the earth. Culturally relevant food also regenerates community members' connection to the land, to a way of life, and to one another. As the Elder Agnes Wesley-Corston stated, getting the youth on the land "to taste the food we used to eat" provides them with a grounding sense of place, values, and belonging as a Cree person. The vitality that has been stripped away by commercial foods is reconstructed through these relationships with the land.

Having skills, access, and mobility to get the food from the land is critical. Food procured through land-based practices does not necessarily make up a large percentage of the diet of many families in Moose Factory. Some of the Cree hunters I interviewed felt that perhaps half of the community was able to secure culturally relevant foods on a semi-regular basis. There are various factors that limit people's accessibility, such as lifestyle changes, mobility, mining development, increasing costs, and administrative demands. Despite these factors, the community continues to find innovative ways of securing local foods. These efforts are motivated by the youth's willingness to learn hunting, fishing, and trapping skills, and the dedication of community leaders like Charlie Cheechoo. These community champions persevere, through the many barriers, to access the significant resources that are needed to run land-based programs and to reconnect generations to the land. With increased reliance on the land for vitality, the shifting notions of food security take on new meanings in these contexts.

Conclusion

When working with Indigenous peoples, we cannot rely on compartmentalized approaches to understanding individual and community well-being. The link between land, culture, food, women, and health in Indigenous communities is evident and well-documented (Adelson 2000; Anderson 2011; Field 2008; Flannery 1995; Palmer 2005; Wilson 2003). All ways of being are interconnected for the people of Moose Cree First Nation. The goal of this chapter is not to make claims about these linkages, nor is it to present a one-dimensional perspective of the Omushekego people's connection to the land. Rather, it is to demonstrate the diverse ways in which the community members are reclaiming their cultural continuance through land-based practices.

External youth programming and funding increased in this community at the time of the 2009 suicide crisis. Such programming was initially focussed on suicide prevention and was often driven by outside organizations that lacked a community-centred exchange of cultural knowledge, in addition to Western approaches to well-being. Yet, through this tragedy, programs expanded to provide land-based skills and knowledge to youth. People started to recognize and to once again reposition Cree knowledge systems as the foundations of youth and community well-being. This recognition and repositioning displaced Western-based approaches, which too often pathologize Indigenous youth, further alienating them from their traditional ways of reconnecting with the land. The land is more than just a physical space. It is an unencumbered space, where the (re)education in the ways of the Elders and the roots of *Pimatisiwin* can be felt and known. Such an understanding allows for a wider lens, reaching beyond land-based programming and local subsistence practices to the broader social contexts of family, community, and local knowledge—land is a site of continuity and empowerment.

The Moose Cree community is entering a new, progressive phase of growth, both economically and socially. The Omushkego people are increasingly assuming control of their own connections to land, as well as of their lives and bodies, and it is important that intrusive outside influences be minimized. The colonial legacy has penetrated the surface of the land with its perverse mechanisms of assimilation and cultural repression. Yet the Omushkego people have a connection to the land that is deeper than the surface. In this context, going back to the land is, in part, remembering that people are an inextricable part of the land. To withstand the ongoing challenges in northern communities, Indigenous peoples are reigniting their sacred fires of knowledge, of history, and of culture. These are their means of counteracting damaging colonial histories, which have been acknowledged in multiple chapters of this book. To renew communities' connections to critical life sources, a greater emphasis on women's contributions and approaches is important. In addition to highlighting the traditional authority and knowledge of women—by discussing their historical roles in restoring connections—this chapter provides insights into specific land-based initiatives that inspire cultural continuance and community well-being. Finally, this chapter emphasizes the importance of long-term investments in community-based initiatives as a means of sustaining the well-being of Omushkego youth.

Notes

1. I give thanks to the Moose Cree community for their hospitality and generosity. It has been an honour to experience the spirit of this land. Moose Cree is a gemstone of a community that is difficult to describe but is incredibly welcoming. I commend their tireless efforts for doing the hard work of safeguarding and preserving that which is sacred to them and to many of us engaged in rebuilding healthy and vibrant communities. This book chapter would be empty without their voices, stories, and knowledge. Special thanks to the visionary women and men who in their hearts hold true the life pathways of an optimistic present and future for their people. I also give thanks to all those who shared their time, enthusiasm, and challenges and also listened to my stories. These collective exchanges weave a tapestry of hope, power, and life for many generations to come.

2. All following direct quotations without page numbers refer to personal interviews conducted by the author of this chapter.

References

Adelson, Naomi. 2000. *"Being Alive Well": Health and the Politics of Cree Well-Being*. Toronto: University of Toronto Press.

Anderson, Kim. 2011. *Life Stages and Native Women: Memory, Teachings, and Story Medicine*. Winnipeg: University of Manitoba Press.

Cheechoo, Charlie. 2014. Personal interview. 13 January.

Cheechoo, Donovan. 2014. Personal interview. 14 January.

Cheechoo, Earl. 2014. Personal interview. 15 January.

Cheechoo, Karen Pine. 2014. Personal interview. 13 January.

Cheechoo, Nathan. 2013. Personal interview. 1 August.

Cheechoo-Linklater, Mary. 2014. Personal interview. 19 March.

Field, Les W. 2008. *Abalone Tales: Collaborative Explorations of Sovereignty and Identity in Native California*. Durham, NC: Duke University Press.

Flannery, Regina. 1995. *Ellen Smallboy: Glimpses of a Cree Woman's Life*. Montreal: McGill-Queen's University Press.

Linklater, Christina. 2014. Personal interview. 19 March.

Linklater, Paul. 2014. Personal interview. 20 March.

Martin, Lawrence. 2014. Personal interview. 13 August.

———. 2015. Personal interview. 10 February.

Palmer, Andie Diane. 2005. *Maps of Experience: The Anchoring of Land to Story in Secwepemc Discourse*. Toronto: University of Toronto Press.

Sailors, Allen. 2014. Personal interview. 17 January.

Shko, Asynee Apay. 2014. Personal interview. 17 March.

Sutherland, Bertha. 2014. Personal interview. 16 January.

Tozer, William. 2014. Personal interview. 19 March.

Wapachee, Kiersten. 2013. Personal interview. 2 August.

Wesley-Corston, Agnes. 2014. Personal interview. 19 March.

Wilson, Kathleen. 2003. "Therapeutic Landscapes and First Nations Peoples: An Exploration of Culture, Health and Place." *Health Place* 9 (2): 83–93.

Conclusion

RESTORING LOCAL
FOOD SYSTEMS

A Call to Action

In *Killing the Shamen* (1985), former Sandy Lake First Nation Chief Thomas Fiddler shares an experience from the 1920s. His story provides an important insight into the dramatic changes Indigenous peoples in Northwestern Ontario experienced as a result of exposure to Euro-Canadian culture and technologies: "In 1925, coming up from Little Grand Rapids, we first saw an outboard motor . . . we saw the prospectors in one canoe, pulling two canoe loads of supplies. . . . We could see these guys just sitting in their canoe, doing nothing. . . . I never forgot that motor. . . . During that winter I collected my pelts and saved them up. I was aiming to get that motor. . . . Immediately, I began the trip back—driving. I didn't work at all. I just sat there" (Fiddler and Stevens 1985, 146–48). Fiddler's account, of witnessing two men effortlessly pull a boat with twice the load, points to the allure of Western technologies and their sudden adoption into Indigenous daily life. This narrative, however, also highlights a series of consequences that emerged as a result of this adaptation. First, Indigenous people became reliant on these new technologies (whether it be iron tools, firearms, or more advanced technologies like outboard engines) to perform everyday tasks. Second, a new unsustainable economic exchange, based on hunting/trapping, came into being and led to an abrupt depletion of critical food and material resources. Third, a new relationship emerged between Indigenous peoples in this region and the newly arrived Euro-Canadians. The growing dependence on Western technologies led to what Ray (1998) refers to as a culture of dependency. The once autonomously thriving Indigenous population become reliant not only on Western technologies, but also on Western economic exchange for survival. These consequences have prompted the writing of this collection and our exploration of how Indigenous people of Northwestern Ontario are striving to move forward from a relationship of dependency toward reclaiming the autonomy their people once knew.

For many communities, this process of reclamation began with restoring connections to the land and by building food capacity from what the land provides. Pre-European contact, it was this intimate relationship with the land that enabled people to live and thrive in this region over millennia. Indigenous people lived semi-nomadically: traversing large tracts of land in small groups and utilizing plant and animal resources to sustain themselves. Knowing how to hunt the vast variety of animal species—they used all parts of the animals for critical food resources and prepared them to optimize their nutritional value—people were able to live in what can be best described as relative abundance (Sahlins 1972). The rapid depletion of these resources and the subsequent change in lifestyles has been a theme throughout this book. Still, how communities are restoring these connections with the land and learning to move forward through local land-based solutions deserves closer attention. Academic research (Willows et al. 2009; Anand et al. 2001) and public reports (Reading and Wein 2009; Health Council of Canada 2005) continue to highlight problems Indigenous peoples in the North are facing, whether it be in terms of poor health, limited resources, high unemployment, substance abuse, food insecurity, or a host of other social and health-related issues. And while people should be aware of the disparities Indigenous peoples are facing, identifying and researching these issues clearly is not enough. Socha et al. (2012) stress this point when writing, "Despite widespread knowledge of the food crisis in remote communities, little attention has been given to community members' suggestions for addressing these problems" (6). For example, the Council of Canadian Academies (2014) brought together an Expert Panel on the State of Knowledge of Food Security in Northern Canada to "seek evidence on the state of knowledge of the factors influencing food security in the Canadian North, and on the health effects of food insecurity among Canada's northern Aboriginal populations" (vii). The panel's report is effective in highlighting the high levels of food insecurity in the North and the complexities of trying to respond to these challenges. It also identifies what it refers to as "promising practices" (local, provincial, territorial, and federal) to improve northern food security. However, the question is at what point will an investment in a panel of research experts, reporting on the concerns northern peoples have been voicing for years, switch to an investment in communities actually trying to address local and regional food access issues? In other words, when will solutions be implemented to address the dire food problems northern Indigenous peoples continue to manage?

The community-based solutions presented in Chapters 3, 4, and 5 are part of a larger movement across Canada where communities and community organizations are attempting to address food challenges through cultural land-based programming. In Nain, Newfoundland and Labrador, a joint project has been established to reconnect youth to the land, as part of a mental wellness strategy, but also to improve local food security (Nain Research Centre 2015). The program Aullak, Sangilivallianginnatuk (Going off, Growing strong) provides young people with the opportunity to learn skills necessary to live off the land. As a pilot project of the Nain Research Centre, the program is "about building connections (social and environmental) and evaluating the success of a community freezer and pilot youth outreach program that aims to enhance the mental, physical, and spiritual health of youth through intensive, long-term engagement and programming" (ibid., para. 3). In Northern Manitoba, Nisichawayasihk Cree Nation (Nelson House First Nation) has developed an off-the-land food program thoroughly documented by Thompson and colleagues (2012). The program builds on traditional food-sharing systems by formalizing the distribution of country foods (foods that are available through hunting/fishing/gathering). The co-authors point out that "Country food sharing, to a lesser degree, occurs in all Aboriginal communities but without community supports and so individuals bear the heavy cost of provisioning" (ibid., 55). Researchers explain that by dedicating resources (financial and human) the Nisichawayasihk community members formalize food-sharing mechanisms and inspire other communities in the region to develop their own food programs. In addition to increasing quality food access for community residents, Thompson and colleagues identify other important contributions this program makes. Their results illustrate how these types of programs provide important socio-economic development for northern communities. The Nisichawayasihk off-the-land project provides "food to 1500 people out of 2500" people in the community and employs local residents to help in the food harvesting, preparation, and distribution (ibid., 54). In addition to the community programs profiled in this book, these are only two examples of local food initiatives that are responding to their community's food crisis and also contributing to its overall health and wellness. Even though some efforts are achieving considerable success by increasing access to nutritious foods, the potential of these programs is even greater when supported by larger government, non-profit, and political organizations. Two programs worth recognizing are the Northern Healthy Foods Initiative (NHFI) in Manitoba and the Remote First Nations Food Systems project (RFNFS) in British Columbia.

In 2002, Manitoba's Healthy Child Committee of Cabinet mandated a Northern Food Prices Project to understand and address the rising food prices in Northern Manitoba (Manitoba Aboriginal and Northern Affairs 2003). Its report identified strategies to reduce costs of healthy market foods, but it also focussed on how to build local food capacity in the North. Three of the seven strategic options put forward specifically targeted building local food autonomy either through food programs, community gardens, or greenhouse developments (ibid.). The NHFI emerged as a result of this report, with the primary aim of supporting local food initiatives (Manitoba Aboriginal and Northern Affairs n.d.). Managed by Aboriginal and Northern Affairs, the NHFI involves provincial departments and agencies working with community-based organizations to assist at a local level. To date, several highly innovative and meaningful initiatives that are contributing to more affordable and more regular access to nutritious foods have received NHFI support. Some of these initiatives include: a beekeeping project in Spence Lake, Barrows, and Meadow Portage; Community Country Food Programs; various agricultural projects tied to greenhouse/nursery developments; and school curriculum and breakfast/ snack programs. An important component to all of these initiatives is social and economic development. From the outset of the Northern Food Prices

Project, it was acknowledged that addressing food security challenges in the North would require multipronged approaches from a diverse array of sectors, and that connecting local food initiatives to social and economic development would be critical. For example, the Ithinto Mechisowin Community Country Food Program "trained: 133 youth; hosted 33 volunteers and worked with nine Elders in the community. Traditional foods were distributed to 126 households creating economic opportunities, through contract employment, for 56 community members and Elders" (Manitoba Aboriginal and Northern Affairs, n.d.). The NHFI approach addresses the complexities of northern food capacity development, focussing not only on improving healthy food access, but also on creating new economic opportunities that will help sustain the programs and create job and training opportunities in the process. The steps that Manitoba is taking to concretely address food insecurity challenges in the North are commendable and its program offers a model from which other provinces could benefit.

British Columbia is also taking appropriate actions to address food challenges in rural remote regions, as evidenced through the RFNFS project developed by the Heart and Stroke Foundation in partnerships with the British Columbia Ministries of Health and Agriculture. The two-year project, funded by the Provincial Health Services Authority, builds on the province's three-year Produce Availability in Remote Communities Initiative. RFNFS provides $700,000 to fifteen Indigenous communities so they can grow their vegetables and fruit. From the outset, the project emphasized community engagement. It involved various stages of in-person dialogue with Elders and community leaders to learn about traditional land-based modes of food procurement, including agricultural practices. Similar to the Northern Healthy Foods Initiative in Manitoba, this project extends beyond gardening and optimizing nutritious food access. To participate, communities are required to develop Agri-Food Plans, integrating local food procurement initiatives within their overall economic development strategies. The plans identify how community food initiatives increase people's access to healthy foods, and outline the steps that ensure the sustainability of their initiatives, whether through external and/or internal funding mechanisms (e.g., small-scale agricultural enterprises). Some communities' garden initiatives are tied into elementary and high school curriculums. They help to teach youth local methods of food procurement, the importance of eating healthy foods, and the potential of gaining control over their food systems in efforts to build local capacity and autonomy. The Agri-Food Plan model is not only important for emphasizing the need to ensure sustainability measures; it properly situates garden initiatives within broader regional food systems, recognizing that gardening is only one avenue toward addressing food insecurity, not a solution unto itself. The RFNFS program has achieved considerable success with relatively limited funding, demonstrating how progressive approaches to food security do not need to involve burdensome investments. The program is currently in its third phase working with funding provided by First Nations Health Authority. In this third phase, the mandate has expanded from working exclusively with rural communities to now working with urban Indigenous populations (organizations and communities) throughout the province.

In the context of Northern Ontario, the Nishnawbe Aski Nation (NAN) is taking the lead in working with communities that are implementing active measures to respond to the growing concerns around Indigenous food security. This region geographically represents approximately two-thirds of Ontario. NAN's mandate is to represent "the legitimate socioeconomic and political aspirations of its First Nation members to all levels of government in order to support local self-determination while establishing spiritual, cultural, social, and economic independence" (NAN 2015). Critical to this self-determination is helping communities regain control over their food systems. Therefore, in 2011, NAN chiefs-in-assembly endorsed "the NAN Food Strategy which outlines 6 key pillars to rebuilding food sovereignty in NAN territory" (NAN 2015b, 6). The progressive strategy being implemented by NAN, under the direction of the NAN Food Sovereignty Committee and with input from NAN communities, focuses on three priority areas: (1) traditional practices, (2) local food production, and (3) imported foods. The strategy is first and foremost a five-year action plan to identify measures that will support these three priority areas. Such measures may include forming collaborative partnerships with government, private enterprise, academia, and non-profit organizations, or securing funding for communities' local food plans. The strategy also involves a series of initiatives that support local food sovereignty efforts in the region. For example, for the past five years NAN has organized and hosted the Annual NAN Food Symposium. This is a knowledge-sharing event where people from all over the region come together to share best practices around local food initiatives, participate in food workshops (e.g., food preparation, cooking, preservation), and celebrate local food traditions. Another example would be Food System Planning—using funding secured through the Ontario Trillium Foundation, NAN worked with ten communities to develop formalized food plans. The food plans enabled communities to control their own food systems by increasing access to nutritious foods and by improving food distribution.

Another level of action orchestrated by NAN, as part of its food strategy, is influencing new modes of land-based food procurement in NAN communities. In 2011, NAN received funding from the Ministry of Health Promotion and Sport to develop what was called the Get Growing Project. The project was designed to promote gardening in select NAN communities to increase the availability and consumption of fresh produce. As outlined in Chapter 3, NAN communities are typically remote and inaccessible by roads, making the shipment of fresh produce expensive and difficult. Fresh produce is rarely available in stores and when it is, it is extremely expensive. The Get Growing Project provided financial support for communities to establish community gardens, but it also offered training to set up gardens, prepare soil, determine what type of fruits and vegetables would optimally grow in the northern environment, and plant seeds and seedlings. Each participating community needed to demonstrate interest, capacity, and willingness to implement some type of gardening activity in their community, but the strength of the program was its flexibility in letting communities determine their own gardening initiatives. In some cases, communities developed centralized gardens; in other communities, backyard gardens were planted in combination with centralized spaces. Some programs involved school children and included gardening and harvesting as part of the school curriculum. The program has been a tremendous success and today these garden initiatives continue to flourish in the pilot communities, as well as in other neighbouring communities that were inspired to also develop gardens and related activities.

The success of the Get Growing Project has also proven inspirational for our Indigenous Health Research Group, and has contributed, in part, to the formation of an ongoing and meaningful partnership with the NAN. As the Get Growing Project was being developed, our group serendipitously received funding from the Public Health Agency of Canada (PHAC) to support garden initiatives in two NAN communities: Wapekeka First Nation and Wawakapewin First Nation. The gardening infrastructure that the communities were able to implement with the resources from the PHAC funding assisted them in successfully applying for the Get Growing Project, which further bolstered their gardening capacity. Our partnership with NAN enabled our research group to work with people like Wendy Trylinski, NAN director of Public Health Education, and Joseph Leblanc, contributor and the past project manager at NAN. They facilitated our learning in regard to working with communities in their efforts toward gaining food sovereignty. The Get Growing Project provided an important model for engaging with Indigenous communities and also revealed the strengths of working collaboratively to address the multifactorial challenges of food security. In fact, this early partnership paved the way for our group's future research projects, ensuring that research objectives and community needs and interests are fully aligned.

This book is an attempt to highlight the important barriers Indigenous communities in Northern Ontario are encountering in getting access to healthy and nutritious foods, and to profile how communities are initiating local land-based strategies to respond to these challenges. However, the collection is also about establishing an approach to working *with* Indigenous communities that brings about the changes required to improve the food system and makes it more historically consistent and culturally meaningful to the people in this region. The NAN Food Strategy helped inform our approach, as did our work with tribal organizations, non-profits, government partners, the communities, and impassioned food actionists.[1] First, our approach acknowledges that there are in fact several approaches to recognizing the diversity of the people and the conditions in which they live. To recognize that these approaches come from within, and are driven by what communities deem essential for their own success, is critical. Perhaps most importantly, these approaches build upon the strengths communities possess, strengths that have been challenged by Euro-Canadian interventions. As argued in Chapter 4, residential schools and the dislocation from land and culture have forever altered Indigenous communities, but a distinct set of skills, values, and traditional knowledges still persevere. By building programs that are land-based and draw from local cultural practices, communities are not simply improving food access, but are engaging in restorative processes that destabilize the relationships of dependency that have influenced Indigenous livelihoods for generations. The efforts that we are celebrating in writing this book are demonstrative of the important steps Indigenous communities are making toward this restorative process. Yet much remains to be done.

There are still several challenges Indigenous peoples face in Northwestern Ontario and access to nutritious foods is simply one of them. At present, communities in this region are under what NAN and the Sioux Lookout First Nations Health Authority are describing as a "state of emergency." They argue that the "unequal access to health care means treatable and preventable diseases are killing people in remote northern communities" (Gignac 2016). This state of emergency was, in part, triggered by a woman dying in the Webequie First Nation because the nursing station ran out of oxygen and could not provide her with the necessary medical attention. This tragic case, however, is only one incident on a long list where people have died unnecessarily due to insufficient health care. The *Globe Mail* reported that in the same region in "2014, a five-year-old boy named Brody Meekis from Sandy Lake First Nation died from strep throat; two four-year-olds—one from Sandy Lake, the other from Pikangikum—died from rheumatic fever" (ibid). Adding to this are other concerns: the alarming increase in suicides, housing shortages and overcrowding, unreasonable living conditions, and lack of access to clean drinking water. It is this combination of factors and tragic events that led NAN to issue a Public Health Emergency "call to the Provincial and Federal governments to commit to a plan of action to begin to address this crisis" (Garrick 2016).

As overwhelming as these problems are, the timing is perhaps ideal to make such a plea for intervention. The new federal government in Canada was elected in 2015, in part, on a campaign that promised "to reset Canada's relationship with its Indigenous people" (Mas 2015). Prime Minister

Trudeau also proclaimed that "It is time for a renewed, nation-to-nation relationship with First Nations peoples, one that understands that the constitutionally guaranteed rights of First Nations in Canada are not an inconvenience but rather a sacred obligation" (ibid.). This same government also promised to act on all ninety-four recommendations of the Truth and Reconciliation Committee (TRC), listed in the report on the residential school system and its enduring legacy on Indigenous peoples throughout Canada. At the conclusion of the report, the prime minister's official statement was: "we will work with leaders of First Nations, Métis Nation, Inuit, provinces and territories, parties to the Indian Residential School Settlement Agreement, and other key partners, to design a national engagement strategy for developing and implementing a national reconciliation framework, informed by the Truth and Reconciliation Commission's recommendations" (Trudeau 2015). At present there is cautious optimism in Canada that the gross (health, socio-economic, etc.) disparities Indigenous peoples are facing will begin to be addressed and that a more respectful relationship between Indigenous peoples and government will be achieved. In response to the health conditions in Northern Ontario, Prime Minister Trudeau stated that he was aware of the crisis and that his government was striving to "fix a relationship that has been broken over the past decade, and indeed centuries, between Canada and Indigenous peoples" (Perkel 2016). The crisis, however, is acute, and while relationship building and addressing larger systemic issues are necessary, this long-term vision must be accompanied with immediate actions to alleviate the immense difficulties communities are facing. Acknowledging that there are serious problems with the health care system and with the level of care the people are receiving in this region is important, but concrete steps need to be taken to provide a level of care that is comparable to that of the rest of the nation.

In this book we have profiled the actions Indigenous communities are taking to address health concerns, by developing local food programs that improve regular access to nutritious foods. But these programs do not function in silos, and without addressing larger health and social issues alongside food security challenges, efforts to improve dietary practices will have little impact. Communities need greater access to clean and safe drinking water. There needs to be a greater investment in housing to address the deplorable living conditions and overcrowding. The education system must be improved so that youth are graduating from high school and receiving postsecondary training. Mental health must become a priority and services need to be put in place for prevention and treatment of related health issues. Law enforcement must resolve the disproportionately high incarceration rates for Indigenous peoples, and provide greater protection to those most vulnerable to violent crime—in particular Indigenous women. The issues are as vast as they are complex, but not insurmountable. Steps toward reconciliation are currently being made and there appears to be a growing spirit to make good on promises that have either been forgotten or ignored by federal, provincial, and territorial governments. What is certain is that we are beyond the point of identifying the issues and their complexities. It is time to invest and put meaningful actions into place.

Notes

1   We borrow this term from the Nishnawbe Aski Nation Food Sovereignty Advisory Group. Often people leading food initiatives in communities are referred to as food champions, but the word "actionist" better captures the tremendous effort and determination required to initiate and sustain the programs being described here.

References

Anand Sonia S., Salim Yusuf, Ruby Jacobs, A.D. Davis, Qilong Yi, H. Gerstein, P.A. Montague, and Eva Lonn. 2001. "Risk Factors, Atherosclerosis, and Cardiovascular Disease among Aboriginal People in Canada: The Study of Health Assessment and Risk Evaluation in Aboriginal Peoples (SHARE-AP)." *Lancet* 358 (9288): 1147–53.

Council of Canadian Academies. 2014. *Aboriginal Food Security in Northern Canada: An Assessment of the State of Knowledge*. Ottawa: The Expert Panel on the State of Knowledge of Food Security in Northern Canada, Council of Canadian Academies.

Fiddler, Thomas, and James R. Stevens. 1985. *Killing the Shamen*. Moonbeam, ON: Penumbra Press.

Garrick, Rick. 2016. "Webequie's Norman Shewaybick Completes 1000 km Walk in Memory of Wife." *Wawatay News*, 3 March.

Gignac, Julien. 2016. "Northern Ontario First Nations Declare Public-Health Emergency." *Globe and Mail*, 24 February.

Health Council of Canada. 2005. *The Health Status of Canada's First Nations, Métis and Inuit Peoples*. Toronto: Health Council of Canada.

Manitoba Aboriginal and Northern Affairs. 2003. *Northern Food Prices Report 2003*. http://www.gov.mb.ca/ana/food_prices/2003report.html.

——. n.d. "Northern Healthy Foods Initiative (NHFI)." http://www.gov.mb.ca/ana/print,nhfi.html.

Mas, Susana. 2015. "Trudeau Lays Out Plan for New Relationship with Indigenous People." *CBC News*, 8 December 2015. http://www.cbc.ca/news/politics/justin-trudeau-afn-indigenous-aboriginal-people-1.3354747.

Nain Research Centre. 2015. "Aullak, Sangilivallianginnatuk (Going Off, Growing Strong)." Nain Research Centre. http://nainresearchcentre.com/research-projects/the-sustainable-communities-initiative/food-security/aullak-sangilivallianginnatuk-going-off-growing-strong/.

NAN (Nishnawbe Aski Nation). 2015. "About Us." http://www.nan.on.ca/article/about-us-3.asp.

Nishnawbe Aski Nation. 2015b. *Reclaiming Our Right to Food Self Determination. Nishnawbe Aski Nation*. Thunder Bay: Nishnawbe Aski Nation.

Perkel, Colin. 2016. "First Nations in 'State of Shock' as They Declare Public-Health Emergency." *TheStar.com*, 24 February. https://beta.thestar.com/news/canada/2016/02/24/first-nations-in-state-of-shock-as-it-declares-public-health-emergency.html.

Ray, Arthur J. 1998. "Periodic Shortages, Native Welfare, and the Hudson's Bay Company, 1670–1930." In *Out of the Background: Readings on Canadian Native History*, edited by Kenneth S. Coates and Robin Fisher. Toronto: Irwin Publishing.

Reading, Charlotte Loppie, and Fred Wien. 2009. *Health Inequalities and Social Determinants of Aboriginal Peoples' Health*. Prince George, BC: National Collaborating Centre for Aboriginal Health.

Sahlins, Marshall David. 1972. *Stone Age Economics*. Chicago: Aldine-Atherton.

Socha, Teresa, Mehdi Zahaf, Lori Chambers, Rawnda Abraham, and Teri Fiddler. 2012. "Food Security in a Northern First Nations Community: An Exploratory Study on Food Availability and Accessibility." *Journal of Aboriginal Health* 8 (2): 5–14.

Thompson, Shirley, Asfia Gulrukh Kamal, Mohammad Ashraful Alam, and Jacinta Wiebe. 2012. "Community Development to Feed the Family in Northern Manitoba Communities: Evaluating Food Activities Based on Their Food Sovereignty, Food Security, and Sustainable Livelihood Outcomes." *Canadian Journal of Nonprofit and Social Economy Research* 3 (2): 43–66.

Trudeau, Justin. 2015. "Statement by Prime Minister on release of the Final Report of the Truth and Reconciliation Commission." *Prime Minister of Canada Justin Trudeau*. http://pm.gc.ca/eng/news/2015/12/15/statement-prime-minister-release-final-report-truth-and-reconciliation-commission#sthash.n1TiChFC.dpuf.

Willows, Noreen D., Paul Veugelers, Kim Raine, and Stefan Kuhle. 2009. "Prevalence and Sociodemographic Risk Factors Related to Household Food Security in Aboriginal Peoples in Canada." *Public Health Nutrition* 12 (8): 1150–56.

Simon Frogg sadly passed away in December of 2016, prior to the release of this book. He was a revered Elder from the Wawakapewin First Nation. He is a founding member of the community, which received band status in 1985 and reserve status in 1998. Wawakapewin (Long Dog in English) is a remote First Nations community approximately 350 kilometres north of Sioux Lookout. It is located on Long Dog Lake and along the southeast shores of the Asheweig River, a tributary of the Winisk River. Simon has been an inspirational leader throughout most of his life, teaching traditional ways and advocating for land-based practices and education. He has served his community and Indigenous peoples throughout Ontario. In his community he has been chief, band manager, elected council member, land-use planning coordinator, Elder, grandfather, father, husband, traditional knowledge keeper, and healer. Outside of his community he has served as the Director of Education with the Ojibway and Cree Cultural Centre, the Vice-President of Northern Nishnawbe Education Council, Treaty Specialist, and Interpreter.

Kristin Burnett is an Associate Professor in the Department of Indigenous Learning at Lakehead University and was recently Lakehead University's Research Chair in Indigenous Health and Well-Being. She is the author of *Taking Medicine: Women's Healing Work and Colonial Contact in Southern Alberta, 1880–1930* (University of British Columbia Press 2010). Burnett's current research project looks at the relationships between health, food sovereignty, and colonialism in northern Indigenous communities. Her work with rural Indigenous peoples is community informed, participatory, and action oriented.

Bénédicte Fontaine-Bisson is an Assistant Professor in the School of Nutrition Sciences at the University of Ottawa and a registered dietitian. She specializes in the field of pregnancy and childhood nutrition. Her research aims to better understand inter-individual variability in response to diet (nutrigenetics) as well as the effect of nutrients on gene expression (nutrigenomics). She combines nutritional and genetic epidemiology approaches to identify genetic, dietary, and environmental factors acting individually or synergistically in the prevention of chronic diseases such as cardiovascular disease, obesity, and type 2 diabetes.

Janice Cindy Gaudet is a Métis researcher and educator from a farming community in Saskatchewan. She is currently an Assistant Professor in the Faculté Saint-Jean, University of Alberta. She is committed to a decolonial approach in research, well-being, and pedagogy by centring Indigenous knowledge. This stems from years of helping Indigenous Elders restore cultural teachings to address social issues. She completed her PhD at the University of Ottawa in the Faculty of Health Sciences. Her research with Moose Cree First Nation in Moose Factory, Ontario, focussed on the importance of land-based knowledge for Omushkego's youth well-being. She currently works as a researcher with DestiNATIONS on a study that highlights Indigenous cultural production in Quebec. She also coordinates a community project with Anishnaabe grandmothers that develops culturally based strategies to prevent human trafficking and sexual exploitation of Anishnabek youth.

François Haman is a biologist who focuses on the relations between food intake, energy metabolism, and the development as well as the treatment of chronic disease. He is a member of the Indigenous Health Research Group at the University of Ottawa and a Full Professor in the School of Human Kinetics. Over the last ten years, he has mostly worked in Northwestern Ontario communities to assess nutritional behaviour, the prevalence of obesity, and type 2 diabetes. His research also helps develop local strategies to improve access to food in northern Indigenous communities.

Benoît Lamarche is Full Professor at the School of Nutrition and Chair of Nutrition at Laval University. He has published more than 270 peer-reviewed papers in areas related to diet and its impact on metabolic syndrome, obesity, inflammation, and dyslipidemia. His research—on the association between small, low-density lipoprotein particles and the risk of coronary heart disease, the effect of trans fat from industrial and ruminant sources on blood lipids, and Mediterranean diets—is highly cited. He has also published work describing the association between diet and cardiometabolic risk factors among Indigenous peoples of Northern Quebec and Ontario. He has contributed to the training of more than fifty graduate students and has received numerous awards, including awards from the Société Québécoise de lipidologie, nutrition et métabolisme (2013 Prix des Fondateurs), the Canadian Nutrition Society (2011 Centrum New Investigator Award), the Utrecht Group and the International Dairy Federation (2004 Wiebe Visser Bi-annual International Nutrition Award). He is also an Olympian (1984, 1988) in long-track speed skating.

Joseph LeBlanc has been engaging in food sovereignty issues for the past decade. He holds an Honours Bachelor of Environmental Studies in Forest Conservation, an Environmental Management Certificate, and a PhD in Forest Sciences from Lakehead University. His community-based-action research explores the relationship between Indigenous food sovereignty and natural resource management in Northern Ontario. He has worked throughout the region, participating in a great diversity of food system initiatives including community and forest gardening, forest and freshwater food systems, community and economic development, food system planning, food assessments, and strategies that support the development of several social enterprises. Joseph is Odawa and a member of the Wiikwemkoong Unceded Territory. As co-chair of Food Secure Canada's Indigenous Circle, he is active in national efforts to create a food strategy for Northern Canada. In 2012, he was awarded a Northwestern Ontario Visionary Award for his actions in building food sovereignty in the region.

Courtney W. Mason worked as a SSHRC Postdoctoral Fellow with the Indigenous Health Research Group at the University of Ottawa where he contributed to community-based food security and health programs in rural Northern Ontario with Oji-Cree peoples and in the Northwest Territories with Dene and Métis communities. He is currently a Canada Research Chair in Rural Livelihoods and Sustainable Communities at Thompson Rivers University in Kamloops, British Columbia. His research examines

how Indigenous communities negotiate pressing health and education issues in the backdrop of enduring colonial legacies. His collaborative research identifies the barriers to and facilitators of local subsistence practices. It focuses on community-driven initiatives that enhance local food
security and tourism development, while supporting cultural continuities.
He is the author of *Spirits of the Rockies: Reasserting an Indigenous Presence
in Banff National Park* (University of Toronto Press 2014).

Shinjini Pilon is an environmental toxicologist working as a Human
Health and Ecological Risk Assessor at Golder Associates. Her past research
expertise focused on the connection between pollutants and human health
impacts, including obesity and type 2 diabetes. With the Indigenous Health
Research Group, she focused on the cost of nutritious foods in rural/remote
Indigenous communities in Northern Ontario and potential exposure to
organic pollutants through the consumption of traditional foods. Shinjini
is also experienced in evaluating trends in toxic algal blooms in rural and
Northern Canada.

Michael A. Robidoux is an award-winning author and Full Professor in
the School of Human Kinetics, University of Ottawa. He researches Indigenous cultural practices as they relate to physical activity and local dietary
practices. He is part of the Indigenous Health Research Group, a multidisciplinary research team representing the fields of Ethnology, Physiology,
Biology, Toxicology, Immunology, and Nutrition Sciences. As a member
of this group, he has led research programs for over ten years investigating
the risk and benefits of land-based food strategies in Northwestern Ontario,
the Northwest Territories, Yukon, and British Columbia. Embracing a participatory research model, he works with rural Indigenous communities in
Northern Canada to help build local food capacity in an effort to provide
regular access to nutritious foods.

Desirée Streit is an Anishinaabe and Métis researcher and educator from
The Pas, a small town in northern Manitoba. Desirée recently completed
her Master of Arts in Education (MAEd) at the University of Ottawa. Her
research focuses on the phenomenon of learning to teach-in-relation and is

informed by a relational, embodied framework centered on the teachings found within the medicine wheel. The work Desirée has done in the past with Indigenous communities and youth, along with her MAEd, inform and inspire her current work as a researcher/policy analyst with the First Nations and Inuit Health Branch of Health Canada. Desirée is committed to connecting with community and to her Anishinaabe culture and continues to do so by taking Anishinaabemowin classes, something she is passing along to her two young sons.